AF289852

Proceedings in Life Sciences

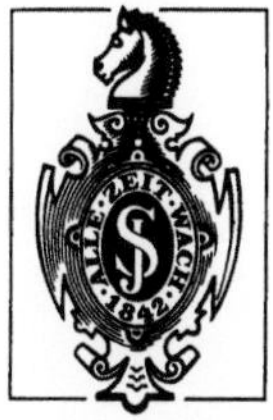

Viral Hepatitis

Edited by
F. Callea, M. Zorzi, and V. J. Desmet

With 12 Figures

Springer-Verlag
Berlin Heidelberg New York
London Paris Tokyo

Dr. Francesco Callea

Aggregaat Hoger Onderwijs, Catholic University of Leuven
Histochemistry Unit, 1st Department of Pathology
Spedali Civili of Brescia, 25100 Brescia, Italy

Professor Dr. Mario Zorzi

Professor of Pathology and Chairman, 1st Department of Pathology
Spedali Civili of Brescia, 25100 Brescia, Italy

Professor Dr. Valeer J. Desmet

Professor of Pathology
Laboratory of Histochemistry and Cytochemistry
Catholic University of Leuven, 3000 Leuven, Belgium

Legend for cover design. Electron microscopic appearance of Delta virus particles isolated from chimpanzee serum. A few 20 nm HBsAg particles are also present. × 175000 (picture by courtesy of Dr. M. G. Canese).

ISBN-13:978-3-642-71352-1   e-ISBN-13:978-3-642-71350-7
DOI: 10.1007/978-3-642-71350-7

Library of Congress Cataloging in Publication Data. Viral hepatitis. (Proceedings in life sciences) Proceedings of the Postgraduate Course on Viral Hepatitis, held in Brescia, Italy in 1985 in honor of the 50th anniversary of the Brescia Division of the Italian Association for Blood donors (AVIS Brescia) Includes index. 1. Hepatitis, Viral–Congresses, I. Callea, F. (Francesco), 1946– . II. Zorzi, M. (Mario), 1920– . III. Desmet, V. IV. Postgraduate Course on Viral Hepatitis (1985: Brescia, Italy) V. Associazione volontari italiani del sangue. Brescia Division. VI. Series. [DNLM: 1. Hepatitis, Viral, Animal–congresses, 2. Hepatitis, Viral, Human–congresses. 3. Hepatitis B Virus–congresses. WC 536 V8128 1985] RC848.H43V56 1986   616.3′623   86-13152

2131/3130-543210

Preface

The Brescia division of the Italian Association of Blood donors (AVIS-Brescia) celebrated its 50th anniversary in 1985. The idea of organizing a Postgraduate Course on Viral Hepatitis on this occasion developed for obvious reasons. Viral hepatitis is a major concern in blood transfusion and Brescia is located in the region of Lombardy characterized by a high HBsAg carrier rate in its population.

Thus it seemed timely to convene a scientific forum in which the present state of knowledge on viral hepatitis would be summarized. This would allow us to review the tremendous progress achieved over the last 15 years, and also to focus on latest developments which pave the way for future investigation.

The publication of the proceedings of this meeting was considered useful, since it provides a tangible reminder of a comprehensive overview of the broad topic of viral hepatitis, its complications, and its connections with the practice of blood transfusion.

The organizers were fortunate in obtaining the active participation of recognized experts in a variety of hepatological disciplines. Their contributions summarized the more mature areas of knowledge in the field, including clinical aspects, epidemiology and morphology, as well as newer developments in the forefront of hepatitis research, like new diagnostic techniques, oncogenesis, treatment, and vaccination.

Therefore we believe that this book will be useful to the busy practitioner in allowing him to find the newest information which otherwise is hidden in a flood of primary literature, and to the specialist in providing a broader framework in which to project his own research efforts.

We are grateful to the speakers and participants for their valuable contributions and thank them for their ready cooperation.

We should like to thank explicitly the AVIS-Brescia, the Assessorato Sanita' and Igiene of the Lombardia Region and Prof. A. Albertini for advice and support, and Springer-Verlag for editing the proceedings.

The Editors

Contents

List of Contributors

You will find the addresses at the beginning of the respective contribution

The Problem of Posttransfusion Hepatitis

F. DEINHARDT[1]

1 Introduction

The problem of posttransfusion hepatitis has changed considerably since the establishment of AVIS 50 years ago. Viral hepatitis has been characterized clinically: the pathology, immunology and virology have been defined, even though much remains to be learned, and this information will be summarized in various chapters of this book (for review see: Vyas et al. 1984). Perhaps the greatest changes in posttransfusion hepatitis have come about primarily by the ability to diagnose hepatitis B virus carriers and secondarily through vaccination against hepatitis B. More change can be expected as the vaccines of the future (prepared by molecular techniques, hybrid viruses or consisting of small synthetic oligopeptides) come into use.

In this brief introduction, I will discuss (1.) the current epidemiological situation, (2.) some experience with recombinant hepatitis B vaccine in healthy adults and in dialysis patients, and (3.) preventive measures against posttransfusion hepatitis.

However, at the outset, it must be understood that not every case of viral hepatitis occurring at the proper interval after blood transfusion is necessarily posttransfusion hepatitis (PTH) caused by hepatits viruses present in the transfused blood (Aach et al. 1978). As an example, Rcinicke (1982) reported several prospective studies of patients undergoing open heart surgery: 30 cases of hepatitis B occurred among 429 patients receiving transfusions (7%) and 13 cases among 151 cases not receiving transfusions or only autologous blood (8.6%). Cases of hepatitis non-A, non-B were not included in these studies. In another study of duodenal ulcer patients treated with truncal vagotomy and pyloroplasty, no hepatitis occurred in 36 patients receiving blood transfusions, and one case of hepatitis non-A, non-B occurred in 49 patients receiving no blood transfusion. These data indicate clearly that despite all precautionary measures, the transmission of hepatitis during ambulatory and/or hospital medical or surgical treatments that do not involve blood transfusions has not been entirely eliminated. It would therefore be incorrect to assume that each case of hepatitis occurring after blood transfusion was caused by the blood transfusion.

1 Max von Pettenkofer Institute for Hygiene and Medical Microbiology, University of Munich, Pettenkoferstr. 9a, 8000 Munich 2, FRG

Viral Hepatitis, ed. by F. Callea et al.
© Springer-Verlag Berlin Heidelberg 1986

2 Viruses Causing Posttransfusion Hepatitis

Several viruses may cause PTH: hepatitis A virus (HAV), hepatitis B virus (HBV), hepatitis delta virus (HDV), hepatitis non-A, non-B viruses (HNANBV), cytomegalovirus (CMV) and Epstein-Barr Virus (EBV) (Aach 1982, Fiedler 1982, Hollinger 1984, Tabor 1985). The distribution of HB and HNANB in several studies is given in Table 1, and the breakdown of CMV, EBV, HAV and HNANBV in cases of hepatitis not caused by HBV is given in Table 2. As can be seen, 91% of all PTH cases are cases of hepatitis non-B, and the majority of these (96%) are caused by the as yet unidentified HNANB viruses.

Hepatitis A has a very short viremic phase, and infection never leads to a chronic virus carrier state. Transmission through blood transfusion, although theoretically possible if blood were to be transfused from a donor during the last days of the incubation period, is extremely rare and plays no practical role. There are very few documented cases of transmission of hepatitis A through blood transfusion.

In more recent studies, less than 10% of PTH is caused by hepatitis B: Its decline to near disappearance as a cause of PTH is due solely to the ability to identify HBV carriers through the detection of HBsAg in the serum, a screening that today's tests for HBsAg have made so sensitive that almost no HBV carriers remain undetected. Theoretically, transmission is possible if blood is donated during the incubation period when HBsAg is still not detectable but when the blood already contains small amounts of infectious HBV. A few cases of chronic, low grade HBV carriers have been reported who were clinically and biochemically undetectable as carriers but who had both circulating

Table 1. Incidence of posttransfusion hepatitis (PTH): Prospective studies

Authors	No. of Patients	Transfused Units/Pat.	Hepatitis	PTH
Reference				
USA	1513	2.4–4.3	171	15 Hepatitis B
TTVS 1981 (4 Centers)			11.3%	156 Hepatitis Non-A, Non-B
Aach et al. 1981			(4%–18%)	91.2%
USA	283	12.7	36	35 Hepatitis Non-A, Non-B
Alter et al. 1981	(Cardiac surgery)		12.7%	97%
West Germany	305	5.6	23	1 Hepatitis B
Sugg et al. 1982	(Cardiac		7.5%	22 Hepatitis Non-A, Non-B
(Univ. Hospital	surgery)			95.6%
Tübingen)				
Australia	842	5.1–6.0	18	3 Hepatitis B
Cossart et al. 1982	(Cardiac		2.1%	1 CMV
(2 Centers)	surgery)			14 Hepatitis Non-A, Non-B
				78%
(from Seidl 1982)				

Table 2. Etiologies of hepatitis non-B following transfusion

Reference	No. hepatitis non-B total hepatitis (% non-B)	Hepatitis A No.	CMV No. (%)[+]	EBV No. (%)[+]	HNANB No. (%)[+]
Cossart et al. 1982	15/18 (78)	0	1[a] (7)	0 –	14 (93)
Tremolada et al. 1982	33/34 (90)	0	3[b] (9)	0 –	30 (91)
Tateda et al. 1979	116/126 (92)	0	0[a] –	0 –	116 (100)
Katchaki et al. 1981	15/18 (78)	0	1[a] (7)	1 (7)	13 (87)
Hollinger et al. 1982	137/151 (91)	0	0[a] –	0 –	137 (100)
Alter et al. 1982	57/61 (94)	0	9[c] (16)	0 –	48 (84)
Total	373/408 (91)	0	14 (3.8)	1 (0.3)	358 (96)

[+] % of all non-B cases
[a] anti-CMV detection by complement fixation (TTVS, only selected cases; Katchaki also by RIA)
[b] anti-CMV detection non-specified
[c] anti-CMV detection by indirect hemagglutination

virus and antibody in their blood even though tests for HBsAg were negative. Testing for anti-HBc titres might identify such individuals because they usually have very high anti-HBc IgG titres and sometimes also anti-HBc IgM titres; however, these cases occur so seldom that extra testing of all blood donations for anti-HBc would be unjustified. Blood is more highly infectious if it contains not only HBsAg and/or HBV DNA. Additional tests for HBsAg and HBV DNA are not recommended for blood donors because the tests are less sensitive than those for HBsAg, they are more expensive, and HBsAg-positive blood must be considered as potentially infectious even when HBeAg and HBV DNA is undetectable.

Hepatitis delta (for review see: Verme et al. 1983) is caused by a defective virus which can only multiply in the presence of HBV; it is not known whether HDV only needs the envelope of HBV to survive outside cells and to be able to infect cells via the cell receptors for HBV, or if HDV also needs HBV for its intracellular replication. Regardless of the mechanism, HDV can only infect and cause hepatitis if exposure to HBV and HDV occurs simultaneously or if a chronic HBV carrier becomes infected with HDV. In the case of infection of an HBV carrier with HDV, very severe forms of hepatitis result. Both the simultaneous primary infection with HBV and HDV, as well as the infection of an HBV carrier, should be excluded by testing all blood donors for HBsAg as almost all HDV-positive bloods also contain detectable amounts of HBV. Nevertheless, severe and fatal cases of hepatitis occur in those parts of the world where testing for HBsAg is insufficient when already debilitated patients become infected with HBV and HDV simultaneously or when HBV carriers become infected with HDV. There is no vaccine or special immunoglobulin available against HDV, but vaccination against HBV also protects indirectly against HDV. Only individuals already infected with HBV remain at risk because HBV vaccines do not terminate or change an HBV carrier state.

The most frequent cause of PTH is hepatitis non A, non B (HNANB) (Hollinger et al. 1981, Tabor and Gerety 1983). Two forms of HNANB have been distinguished: the orally and the parenterally transmitted forms of the disease. The orally transmitted disease has many similarities with HA, and, although not shown conclusively, disease is probably caused by a picornavirus (Purcell et al. 1982). The disease spreads by contaminated water and food supplies as well as by other faecal-oral transmissions associated with poor hygiene. Like hepatitis A, it probably has only a short viremic phase, and transmission via transfusion of blood or blood products has not been reported. Parenterally transmitted HNANB tends to become chronic even more frequently (up to 40–60%) than hepatitis B, but it also appears to resolve by itself more frequently after some years. The persistence of a carrier state over many years has been established by transmission from the same donor over prolonged periods of time to various recipients of blood transfusion. Today, this form of hepatitis is the most frequent type of PTH. A specific exclusion of HNANB virus carriers from donor panels remains impossible because the causative agents have not been identified, and no tests have been developed to diagnose a carrier state.

Cytomegalovirus (CMV) is the second most frequent cause of PTH after HBV and is responsible for 0–16% of PTH in various studies (Table 2). These widely different incidences of CMV-PTH may be due partly to inadequate diagnosis in some studies, but they may also be due to differences in the population groups. In general, CMV probably accounts for 5–10% of all PTH. Immunosuppressed patients without antibodies to CMV are particularly at risk of developing serious posttransfusion CMV infections, and these patients should only receive blood from CMV-free donors. Inoculation of larger amounts of immunoglobulins with high antibody titers against CMV (anti-CMV) has been advocated if CMV-free blood is not available for transfusion, or if the immune status of an immunosuppressed recipient is unknown. The results of such prophylaxis with high titered anti-CMV immunoglobulins have varied, and such recommendations are still under debate.

Epstein-Barr virus may also cause PTH, together with a generalised disease similar to the infectious mononucleosis occurring after natural EBV infections. It would be preferable to use EBV-free blood for immunosuppressed patients, but the very high incidence for EBV infections in the general population, and the probable life-long carrier state after a primary EBV infection, make this very difficult to achieve.

3 Vaccination Against Viral Hepatitis

Vaccination against hepatitis A is in the early stages of development: live attenuated, inactivated whole virus, and recombinant or synthetic oligopeptide vaccine preparations are under study. These vaccines will be of general public health importance but will not influence PTH.

The plasma-derived HBsAg hepatitis B vaccine has been shown to be absolutely safe, highly efficacious and free of major side reactions. However, the vaccine is not sufficiently immunogenic in immunosuppressed individuals such as dialysis patients, and the vaccine is expensive. Its source (HBsAg-containing human plasma) is limited and will become increasingly so in future. Attempts have been made, therefore, to prepare HBsAg by molecular techniques: the entire genome of HBV has been cloned, mapped and sequenced, thus making it possible to identify the genome regions coding for

HBsAg. These genome fragments can be cut out of the genome, amplified in plasmids in bacteria, and used to produce HBsAg in an expression system such as yeast cells. Use of mammalian cells as expression systems for the production of HBsAg has also been discussed: the cost and potential contamination of primary cells with other viruses, and the potential neoplastic characteristics of established cell lines carrying oncogenes, make these cells generally unacceptable. Vaccines prepared in such cells may become acceptable once ways of production are developed that exclude all possible harmful nucleic acid or protein contamination. The experience with recombinant hepatitis B vaccines prepared in yeast has been summarized recently (for review see: Vyas et al. 1984) and the results obtained by various groups of investigators were very similar. In our own studies with the recombinant hepatitis B vaccine (prepared in yeast by the Merck Sharp & Dohme Research Laboratories, West Point, PA, USA), seroconversion rates and antibody titres (anti-HBs) were comparable to results previously obtained with plasma-derived vaccines, with the exception that antibody rises occurred somewhat but insignificantly later than after vaccination with plasma-derived vaccine (Jilg et al. 1984, 1985; Jilg and Deinhardt 1986). The vaccine was free of major side reactions, and minor reactions were similar in frequency and severity to the reactions observed after use of plasma-derived vaccine; i.e., short term swelling, itching and reddening of the injection site and a low grade fever, that however, also occurred with a similar frequency in non-vaccinated controls.

Results of vaccination of healthy adults with the recombinant vaccine prepared in yeast cells by the Merck Sharp and Dohme Research Laboratories are given in Figs. 1 and 2 and of dialysis patients in Fig. 3. As can be seen, high seroconversion rates and

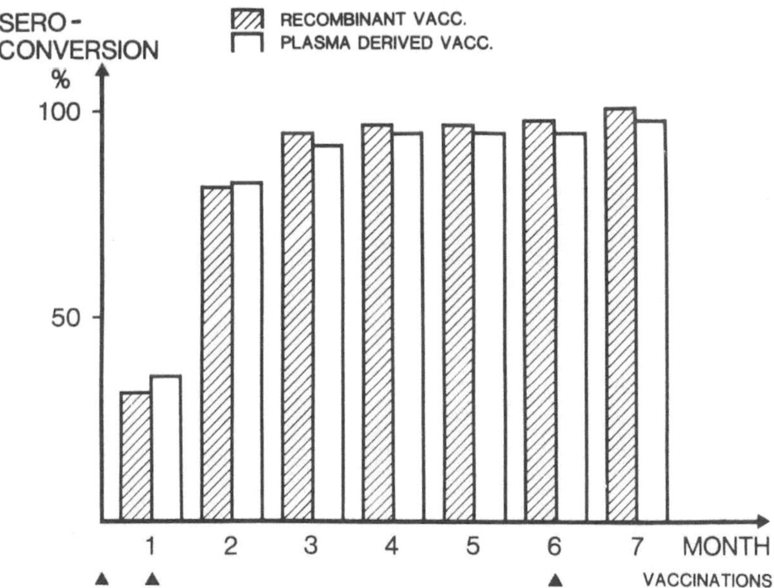

Fig. 1. Seroconversion rates after vaccination with recombinant or plasma-derived hepatitis B vaccine. 10 µgr of HBsAg was given at 0, 1 and 6 months (Jilg and Deinhardt 1986)

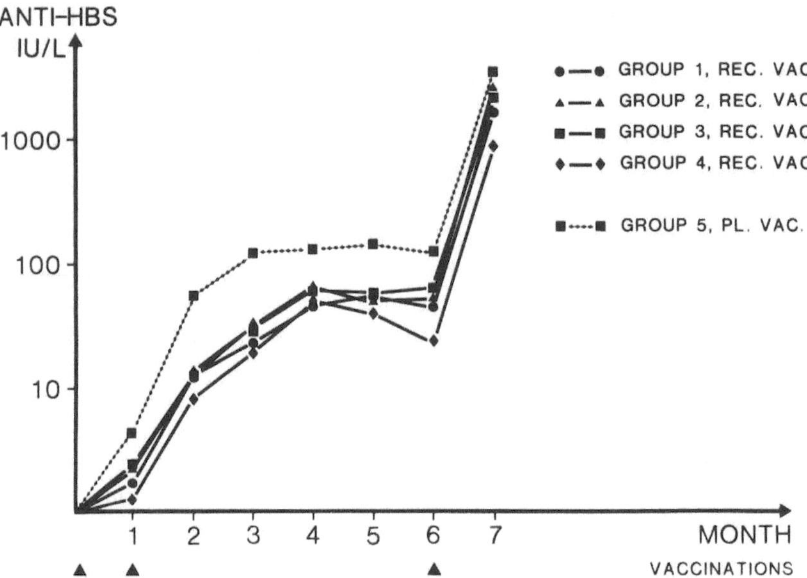

Fig. 2. Comparison of recombinant and plasma-derived hepatitis B vaccine. 10 µgr of HBsAg was given at 0, 1 and 6 months. Groups 1–4 received different lots of recombinant vaccine and group 5 plasma-derived vaccine (Jilg and Deinhardt 1986)

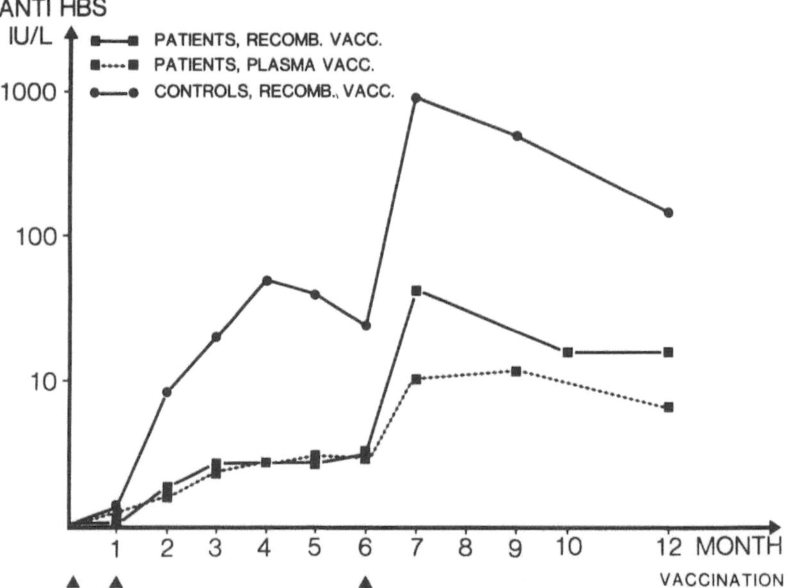

Fig. 3. Anti-HBs responses (geometric mean anti-HBs concentration, all subjects) of dialysis patients (n=49) and healthy controls (n=16) after vaccination with recombinant hepatitis B vaccine, and of dialysis patients after vaccination with plasma-derived vaccine (n=75). 40 µgr HBsAg per dose were given at 0, 1 and 6 months to patients, and 10 µgr HBsAg at the same schedule to controls (Jilg and Deinhardt 1986)

adequate antibody titres were achieved in healthy young adults, but only 60% seroconversion and lower anti-HBs levels in dialysis patients. The response of dialysis patients to the recombinant vaccine was slightly better than to the plasma-derived vaccine, but this difference was statistically insignificant and does not solve the problem of the lack of efficient immunization of all dialysis or other immunosuppressed patients. Preliminary data also indicate that the recombinant vaccine can be used safely and effectively in newborns, with or without simultaneous inoculation of hepatitis B immunoglobulin (HBIG) (Stevens 1986). Vaccination is recommended for all groups at risk of infection with HBV, particularly newborns of HBV carrier mothers, medical and dental personnel, dialysis patients, patients with hemophilia or patients before major operations during which blood transfusions can be foreseen. In the future, if broader vaccination programs can be instituted in high incidence areas for hepatitis B, this disease may be completely eradicated.

No immunoprophylactic measures either in form of specific immunoglobulins or of vaccines are available for HNANB because the causative agents are unknown, and vaccines against CMV and EBV are not yet available or are still in the development.

4 Prevention of Posttransfusion Hepatitis

Exclusion of HBV carriers as blood donors through testing for HBsAg has become routine and needs no further discussion here. In addition to testing for HBsAg, testing serum alanine aminotransferase (ALT) levels of all blood donations has also been recommended as a means of preventing about 1/3 of all PTH, including HNANB (Seidl 1982). Testing for ALT has been discussed frequently on both sides of the Atlantic, and opinions for and against the cost-effectiveness of this test have been argued vehemently (Aach et al. 1978; Hollinger 1984). My own opinion is that ALT testing does provide extra safety, and it should be performed whenever possible. Even though unimportant for preventing hepatitis, all blood donations should be tested also for antibodies against LAV/HTLV III to exclude carriers of this virus, the cause of AIDS.

In general, donations from genuinely voluntary blood donors transmit all forms of PTH less frequently than do those from commercial blood donors: if possible, only voluntary blood should be used. Individuals belonging to risk groups for LAV/HTLV III infections also carry a higher risk of infections with hepatitis viruses: such risk groups include homosexuals, drug addicts, prostitutes, and sexual partners of these groups. In the past, hemophilia patients were another risk group, although their disease prevented them being blood donors.

Transfusion of "warm blood" should be discouraged, and only blood which has been tested for HBsAg and anti-LAV/HTLV III should be used. If "warm blood" transfusions are unavoidable, a donor panel should be assembled that is tested regularly and is composed of individuals who can be assumed not to belong to a risk group. Blood products, such as clotting factors (factor VIII and IX), which carry the risk of transmitting hepatitis and/or LAV/HTLV III should be inactivated (heat of β-propiolactone in combination with UV) (Hollinger 1984).

Last but not least, blood transfusions should be given only when really necessary. Even today, blood transfusions are given unnecessarily, often without weighing possible benefit against the unavoidable risks. It is probably true that most single unit blood transfusions are unnecessary, and evaluation of their frequency in a particular setting indicates the stringency with which decisions to transfuse are handled.

All of the above measures will reduce the incidence of PTH, but control of this problem will become possible only after the agents of HNANB have been identified and characterized, and after tests have been developed to identify HNANBV carriers. Control of the much smaller numbers of PTH caused by CMV and EBV must wait until effective vaccines for general use against these viruses have been developed and appropriate vaccination programs have been implemented.

References

Aach RD, Lander JJ, Sherman LA, Miller WV, Kahn RA, Gitnick GL, Hollinger FB, Werch C, Szmuness W, Stevens CE, Kellner A, Weiner JM, Mosley JW (1978) Transfusion transmitted viruses: interim analysis of hepatitis among transfused and non-transfused patients. In: Vyas GN, Cohen SM, Schmid R (eds) Viral hepatitis. Franklin Inst Press, Philadelphia, pp 383–396

Aach RD, Szmuness W, Mosley JW, Hollinger FB, Kahn RA, Steven CE, Edwards VM, Werch J (1981) Serum alanine aminotransferase of donors in relation to the risk of Non-A, Non-B hepatitis in recipients: The transfusion-transmitted viruses study. N Engl J Med 304: 989–994

Aach RD (1982) Transfusion associated hepatitis: an overview. In: Overby L, Deinhardt F, Deinhardt J (eds) Viral hepatitis: 2nd Int Max von Pettenkofer Symp. Dekker, New York Basel, pp 217–223

Alter HJ, Purcell RH, Holland PV, Alling DW, Koziol DE (1981) Donor transaminase and recipient hepatitis. Impact on blood transfusion services. J Am Med Assoc 246: 630–634

Alter HJ, Purcell RH, Feinstone SM, Tegtmeier GE (1982) Non-A, Non-B hepatitis: its relationship to cytomegalovirus, to chronic hepatitis and to direct and indirect test methods. In: Szmuness W, Alter HJ, Manyard JE (eds) Viral hepatitis, 1981 Int Symp. Franklin Inst Press, Philadelphia, pp 279–294

Cossart YE, Kirsch S, Ismay SL (1982) Post-transfusion hepatitis in Australia. Report Aust Red Cross study. Lancet i: 208–231

Fiedler H (1982) Transfusion associated hepatitis workshop in viral hepatitis. In: Szmuness W, Alter HJ, Maynard JE (eds) Viral hepatitis, 1981 Int Symp. Franklin Inst Press, Philadelphia, p 815

Hollinger FB (1984) Prevention of posttransfusion hepatitis. In: Vyas GN, Dienstag JL, Hoofnagle JH (eds) Viral hepatitis and liver disease. Grune and Stratton, Orlando, pp 319–337

Hollinger FB, Alter HJ, Holland PV, Aach RD (1981) Non-A, Non-B posttransfusion hepatitis in the United States. In: Gerety RJ (ed) Non-A, Non-B hepatitis. Academic Press, New York London, pp 49–70

Hollinger FB, Mosley JM, Szmuness W, Aach RD, Melnick JL, Afifi A, Stevens CE, Kahn RA (1982) Non-A, Non-B hepatitis following blood transfusion: risk factors associated with donor characteristics. In: Szmuness W, Alter HJ, Maynard JE (eds) Viral hepatitis, 1981 Int Symp. Franklin Inst Press, Philadelphia, pp 361–376

Jilg W, Deinhardt F (1986) Results of immunization with a recombinant yeast-derived hepatitis B vaccine. J Infection (in press)

Jilg W, Schmidt M, Zoulek G, Lorbeer B, Wilske B, Deinhardt F (1984) Clinical evaluation of a recombinant hepatitis B vaccine. Lancet ii: 1174–1175

Jilg W, Schmidt M, Weinel B, Küttler TH, Brass H, Bommer J, Müller R, Schulte B, Schwarzbeck A, Deinhardt F (1986) Immunogenicity of recombinant hepatitis B vaccine in dialysis patients. J Hepatology (in press)

Katchaki JN, Siem TH, Brower R, van Loon A, van der Logt JTH (1981) Posttransfusion hepatitis in the Netherlands. Br Med J 282: 107

Purcell RH, Pavri K, Dienes H, Kamimura T, Popper H (1982) Epidemic non-A, non-B hepatitis. In: Overby LR, Deinhardt F, Deinhardt J (eds) Viral hepatitis: 2nd Int Max von Pettenkofer Symp. Dekker, New York Basel, pp 31–34

Reinicke V (1982) Hepatitis in blood transfused patients. In: Overby LR, Deinhardt F, Deinhardt J (eds) Viral hepatitis: 2nd Int Max von Pettenkofer Symp. Dekker, New York Basel, pp 229–233

Seidl S (1982) Hepatitis associated with transfusion and substitution therapy: an introduction. In: Overby LR, Deinhardt F, Deinhardt J (eds) Viral hepatitis: 2nd Int Max von Pettenkofer Symp. Dekker, New York Basel, pp 213–216

Stevens C (1986) Perinatal hepatitis B virus transmission: Prevention with HBIG and recombinant hepatitis B vaccine. In: Seah CS, Zuckerman AJ (eds) Ann Acad Med Singapore (in press)

Sugg U, Erhardt S, Lissner R, Schneider E (1982) ISH/ISBT Congress Budapest

Tabor E (1985) Infections transmitted by blood transfusion. In: Das PC et al (eds) Supportive therapy in haematology. Nijhoff, Boston Dordrecht Lancaster, pp 307–317

Tabor E, Gerety RJ (1983) The agents of Non-A, Non-B hepatitis. In: Deinhardt F, Deinhardt J (eds) Viral hepatitis: Laboratory and clinical science. Dekker, New York Basel, pp 117–137

Tateda A, Kikucki K, Numazaki Y, Shirachi R, Ishida N (1979) Non-B hepatitis in Japanese recipients of blood transfusions: clinical and serologic studies after the introduction of laboratory screening of donor blood for hepatitis B surface antigen. J Inf Dis 139: 511

Tremolada F, Realdi G, Noventa F, Alberti A, Pornada E, Valfre C, Galluci V (1982) Post-transfusion hepatitis in Italy. Lancet i: 853–854

Verme G, Bonino F, Rizzetto M (1983) Viral hepatitis and delta infection. Liss, New York

Vyas GN, Dienstag JL, Hoofnagle JH (1984) Viral hepatitis and liver disease. Grune and Stratton, Orlando London

Clinical Aspects of Acute and Chronic Hepatitis: Pitfalls of Diagnosis, Extrahepatic Manifestations and Prognosis of the Chronic Disease

J. DE GROOTE[1]

1 Introduction

The usual clinical aspects of acute and chronic hepatitis are well-known phenomena which will not be described at length in this limited review. It seems, however, worthwhile to discuss less common problems and pitfalls of diagnosis. Moreover, attention will also be focused on the spectrum of extrahepatic clinical manifestation, which may also be present as symptoms and obscure the diagnosis, or as complications and endanger the outlook for the patient. The intriguing problem of the evolution and prognosis of acute and chronic hepatitis will be discussed in the last section.

2 Problems and Pitfalls of Diagnosis

It may seem easy to diagnose acute hepatitis; in fact, it often happens that the patient himself says to the doctor "I look yellow: what about my liver? or what about hepatitis?". The initial symptoms are usually atypical and mostly described as "flu-like".

Many cases of hepatitis may not be apparent; how many is very difficult to tell. A French clinical study revealed only 5% cases of overt acute hepatitis in a population which was 75% anti-HAV-positive (Soulier et al. 1978). About the same figure was obtained for HBV hepatitis (Benhamou 1979).

For hepatitis NANB it is known that half of the posttransfusional cases remain asymptomatic; the figure for the sporadic ones is totally unknown.

In hepatitis A, the starting of disease is more abrupt: 60% of the patients describe the transition period as very short and happening within 24 h. The classical prodromal symptom, fatigue, lasts usually only a few days (Krikler 1971).

Hepatitis B is known to have an incubation time of several months. The prodromal period with the vague "flu-like" symptoms and the annoying fatigue is remembered by the patient as a weeks-long trouble, often wrongly ascribed to other causes, especially psycho-social ones. The transition to jaundice is slow and inconspicuous. It has also been described that in volunteers an incubation syndrome appeared within about 50 days after inoculation, consisting of headache, loss of appetite, nausea, and occasionally vomiting. These mild symptoms lasted only a few days but were accompanied by a

---

1 Department of Hepatology, Internal Medicine, Universitaire Ziekenhuis,
St-Rapäel-Gasthuisberg, Herestraat 49, 3000 Leuven, Belgium

slight rise of transaminases. After this the patient was usually well until the outbreak of the major disease (Neefe et al. 1944).

In NANB hepatitis the clinical prodromal state seems to be more variable. The disease starts either abruptly or more insidiously. The transition is also not uniform, but the fatigue is more pronounced. The symptomatology of the acute disease is usually not so intense and resembles more the HBV hepatitis. In the Far East and also North Africa, a completely different form of water-borne epidemic NANB hepatitis has been described, which appears to be very abrupt at the beginning. The disease is also characterized by higher mortality in pregnant women (Khuroo et al. 1981).

The clinical features of a HDV infection are mixed with those of a HBV-positive disease. In most cases an exacerbation of the original disease is witnessed. If the acute disease is due to a simultaneous HBV and HDV infection, more cases with a severe course, even with fulminant liver necrosis, will be observed.

The classical liver tests are of great help in the diagnosis of hepatitis. Nevertheless, they are never pathognomonic for a particular disease. High transaminases are perhaps more in favour of hepatitis; it should be realized that in a clearcut case of obstruction, as ascertained by surgery and biopsy, they may exceptionally rise to 800 IU/l, values up to 400 IU/l are very usual. Moreover transaminases may be rather low (less than 100 IU/1) in cases of cholestatic hepatitis either viral or drug-induced (e.g., phenothiazine) or even normal in cases of pure cholestasis due to alkylated steroids. With the advent of echograpy and CT-scan, ERCP, and PTC, it became much easier to differentiate quickly between cholestasis due to cellular or small duct pathology and large obstruction.

Case A. 53 years. This patient had several bouts of vague abdominal pain and the classical liver test showed increased values. A biopsy showed aspecific lesions.

He was seen by us for the first time as an outpatient for a general check-up. He had no complaints at all. The clinical examination and liver tests were perfectly normal.

During the night he developed severe pain in the right hypochondrium, which was diagnosed as a biliary colic. The presence of lithiasis was confirmed by echography. A cholecystectomy was performed and a stone was extracted from the choledochus.

	Bilirubin	GOT	GPT	Alk. Phosph.	GGT
Previous	1.2	74	78	205	168
Day 1. – outpatient	0.8	10	14	107	21
Day 2. – after colic	1.0	175	182	140	42
Day 3.	1.7	160	140	210	120
Day 4. – post-Op.	1.4	84	46	160	40
Later	0.8	16	18	120	47
Nl.	1 mg/dl	< 19U/l	< 24U/l	< 140U/l	< 22U/l

Case B. 80 years. This lady was a missionary in the tropics for many years. She has mild hypertension and suffers occasionally from angina pectoris. A few days prior to observation, jaundice and dark urine without symptome were observed. Clinical examination was irrelevant except for a palpable liver, 3 cm below the costal margin.

Medication: atenolol, isosorbide, dihydroergotamine. Liver tests: bilirubin 16 mg/dl, GOT 594 U/l, GPT 554 U/l, Alk. Phosph. 316 U/l, GGT 130 U/l. Viral markers: anti HBS > 125U, anti-HAV +. Echography: liver, bile ducts, and pancreas normal. Liver biopsy: acute hepatitis, viral type.

3 Extrahepatic Manifestations

The importance of considering the extrahepatic symptoms in hepatitis stems from the consideration that they are the expression of a physio-pathological process other than the liver symptoms. Of course both depend on the introduction of the virus into the body and the reaction of the immunological system.

The extrahepatic pathology is due to damage in other tissues which may occur without liver trouble. It may preceed the liver disease and be observed as the presenting symptom. It may even become apparent after the liver disease. Most of the extrahepatic manifestations described during the course of an acute hepatitis resemble the serum sickness syndrome. It is known that in this syndrome circulating immune complexes (CIC) are important in the pathogenesis of arthritis, angioedema, and rash (Dixon et al. 1958). It was therefore logical to assume a similar pathogenesis. Several studies seem to confirm this hypothesis (Wands et al. 1975). It is known that immune complexes circulate in acute as well as in chronic hepatitis. They are, however, not found in patients without extrahepatic complaints. Most authors observed about 75% of acute B-hepatitis patients positive for CIC. These complexes disappear with the resolution of the disease. In chronic hepatitis these figures vary between 25% and almost 90%. In chronic carriers CIC-positive are much less frequent, between 0% and about 20%. In most cases the classical and alternative pathway of the complement is activated.

Periarteritis nodosa (PAN) and glomerulonephritis are also related to HBV (NANB) and CIC. Glomerular deposits of HB antigens and immunoglobulins have been observed in renal biopsy specimens in up to one third of the cases in some series. The presumed hepatic disease could be not apparent. The incidence in PAN may be even higher and varies from 31% to 69%. The HBsAg was demonstrated within the vessel wall of the affected artery. The relationship with clinical hepatitis is obscure: overt hepatitis seldom appeared in a patient with HBV-positive PAN.

The pathogenesis of these lesions still remains obscure. It is not known why in some cases an impressive liver necrosis takes place and why in others the liver remains intact, but the arteries or some other tissue suffer. The local situation seems to be regulatory, but this is largely unknown. Several possibilities have been put forward, such as complement binding, vasoactive substances, activation, or depression of T- and B-lymphocytes (Cochrane and Hawkins 1968). Van Damme (1977) suggested the hypothesis that especially the local formation of immune complexes produced toxic lesions.

3.1 Dermatologic Manifestations

Pruritus is a frequent symptom in hepatitis as well as in biliary obstruction; it is probably due to the deposition of bile salts in the skin and should not be considered as an extrahepatic manifestation as such. It is a consequence of the liver disturbance itself.

Dermatologic manifestations are common in hepatitis. Often the skin lesion is due to an urticarial eruption which may be diffused or localized or have the aspect of Quincke's angioedema with swelling of the lips and eyelids. It may be observed as the first manifestation of the disease (Jongedyk-Brondsted et al. 1980). Many other lesions have been described: erythematous (sometimes scarla-like) maculo-papular eruption, acnea, erythematous noduli and purpura-like eruptions without thrombopenia or otherwise disturbed coagulation. The urticaria rarely lasts more than 1 week. It appears in 17% of hepatitis non-B patients and in 38% of HBV-positive ones. These troubles arise in the pre-icteric and often appear together with the joint symptoms (Stewart et al. 1978). These lesions are due to the deposition in the derma of immune complexes, as has been shown by immunofluorescence (Weiss et al. 1978). They are also accompanied by a decrease in serum complement.

A particular cutaneous lesion may affect children of less than 10 years old (Gianotti 1973, 1978). It is the infantile papulous acrodermatitis or syndrome of Gianotti-Crosti, and is very rare in adults (Claudy et al. 1977). The lesions consist of small papules of 1–3 mm diameter, which are dark red, sometimes even purple. They appear on the face, neck, and members and are distributed in a roughly symmetrical fashion. They seem to begin all at once and last for about 3–6 weeks. This syndrome may be accompanied by adenopathy. The liver disease is mostly anicteric and mild, but the children often become HBsAg carriers (Colombo et al. 1977). The Gianotti-Crosti syndrome can be produced by other causes, although hepatitis is the most frequent one. The pathogenesis of this syndrome is also attributed to a deposition of immune complexes, although Gianotti (1978) has doubts about its origin.

Muscular Pain. Muscular pain (myalgia) is very common in the prodromal and/or pre-icteric period of hepatitis. It is often not due to an inflammatory myositis: the serum creatine-phosphokinase is not elevated as it is leptospirosis (Johnson et al. 1975). The cause of the muscular pain is less clear, but it could be due to an arteriolar disturbance.

Real myositis and polymyositis may occur in hepatitis B, but this is exceptional. This complication is accompanied by very severe muscular pain and is diagnosed by an elevation of the serum creatine-phosphokinase. This syndrome is also attributed to the deposition of immune complexes in the muscualr tissue (Michas et al. 1975). Bacon and coworkers (1975) examined 13 patients with polymyalgia rheumatica for evidence of HBV infection. Nine of them were anti-HBs-positive. In view of this association, polymyalgia rheumatica may represent an abnormal immunological response, among others to HBsAg in the elderly patient.

Joint Symptoms. The joint symptoms present themselves most commonly as simple arthralgias, more or less symmetrical. They are frequently localized at the small articulations of the hand and the wrist. In about 10% of the patients these joints are swollen, warm, and red (Onion et al. 1971; Fernandez and McCarty 1971; Schumacher and Gall 1974). In some patients these symptoms represent the only complaint of a subclinical hepatitis which is mostly HBV + (Stevens et al. 1972). The joint pain appears mostly in the prodromal period and disappears usually when the patient becomes jaundiced. The complaint may be short-lived, but can last for a long time and even persist after the clinical cure and normalization of liver tests. Frank arthritis is less common and occurs in a small proportion (1%) hepatitis-B positive cases.

The frequency of the joint symptoms has been variably observed in the past. However, when attention is focused on them, it may be observed in about one third of the patients and even more in elderly ones (Stewart et al. 1978).

Vascular Lesions. Necrotizing vasculitis may develop in a few patients either during or after an acute HBV-positive hepatitis (Drueke et al. 1980). These lesions resemble those of hypersensitivity angiitis or polyarteritis nodosa (PAN) (Sergent et al. 1976; McIntosch et al. 1976). The same distrubances have been observed in chronic HBV-positive cases. The appearance of the PAN vasculitis type lesions are certainly related in some way to the presence of the HB virus. However, the severity of liver lesions do not seem to be in relationship with the vascular pathology. The hepatitis may be mild, subclinical, or even totally inapparent. In one series only 6% of the patients had abnormal liver tests (Mowrey and Lundberg 1954). The frequency of this type of lesion is difficult to evaluate because of the discrepancy between the hepatic and the arterial pathology. The HB virus etiology accounts for 20–50% of all PAN cases (Trepo and Thivolet 1970; Gocke et al. 1970; Duffy et al. 1976). Immunofluorescent microscopy has shown the presence of HBsAg, anti-HBs and immunocomplexes in the arterial lesions (Fye et al. 1977). A cause-effect relationship is generally accepted.

Hypersensitive vasculitis and deposition of cryoglobulins are rare findings in HBsAg+ hepatitis (Sergent et al. 1976; McIntosh et al. 1976). The relationship of the so-called essential form of cryoglobulinemia and the presence of the HB virus remains controversial. In a study of this problem by Popp and co-workers (1980), evidence of HBV markers was detected in about one third of the cryoprecipitates from patients with the underlying HBV disease and in only 10% of those with the essential form. Levo et al. (1977) found HBV viral particles in 4 out of 30 patients, but more often HBsAg or the antibody. Liver tests were abnormal in 26 of them. These patients complained of purpura, arthralgia, and also had renal abnormalities.

Cosgriff and Arnold (1977) described an exceptional case of the Raynaud phenomenon with severe digital vasospasm followed by an infarction of the finger tips and also considerable pain.

Glomerular Lesions. Kidney lesions, especially in the glomeruli, with functional disturbances are rarely observed in acute hepatitis (Conrad et al. 1964). Wilkinson and co-workers (1978) described cases of renal failure in otherwise uncomplicated acute viral hepatitis.

Glomerular lesions are much more frequent in chronic hepatitis and liver cirrhosis. Their co-existence was described as early as 1946 by Baxter and Asworth. More recently, a relationship with the HBV has been demonstrated (Patek et al. 1951; Combes et al. 1971; Knieser et al. 1974). Focal glomerulonephritis was produced in baboons after inoculation with HBsAg-containing plasma (Gyorkey et al. 1975). In about half of the clinical cases studied, the glomeruli contained HBV markers (Ray 1979; Brzosko et al. 1974). The characteristic granular deposition of the HBsAg in the mesangium and/or in capillary walls and also the presence of complement and immunoglobulins suggests the formation and deposition of HBsAg immunocomplexes in the glomerulus, and hence lesions due to their presence. Several histologic types of glomerular lesion, have been observed. The specific role of viral antigen and the circumstances leading to a particular type of lesion should be further documented. This disturbance could be related to the Berger disease (Berger and Hinglais 1968).

Knecht and Chisari (1978) described a remarkable case with glomerular lesions, which regressed after the disappearance of the HB virus. In a group of 101 cirrhotic patients, we observed microscopic hematuria and slight proteinuria. These findings could be interpreted in about one third as the first sign of an otherwise inapparent glomerular lesion. The glomerular pathology progressed in 6 patients, to a frank proteinuria and even to a nephrotic syndrome with intractable, massive ascites, and oedema (De Groote et al. 1980).

Pleuritis and Pericarditis. Pleuritis and pericarditis are findings during hepatitis. They are often associated (Di Matteo et al. 1964; Laverdant et al. 1965; Gross and Gerding 1971; Owen and Shapiro 1974). Pleuritis should be differentiated from pleural effusion, which occurs when ascitic fluid escapes through small openings in the diaphragma.

Pleuritis occurs sometimes in association with cutaneous and articular lesions. It is most often observed in the pre-icteric period of the hepatitis. Whenever HBV was investigated, it proved to be positive (Owen and Shapiro 1974). Pleuritis should be suspected when the patient complains of severe thoracic pain worsened by respiration. Dispnoea on exertion and other symptoms of cardiac tamponade suggest pericarditis. Circulating immune complexes have also been incriminated as cause of this complication.

Neurological Manifestations. Neurological manifestations can occur during hepatitis. Simple peripheral neuritis has been described and proven by conduction studies (Davison et al. 1972; Apstein and Koff 1979). This complication occurs most often late in a HBV+ disease. The lesions regress when the hepatitis improves. It is doubted if they are related to the immune complex disorders.

Neuropathy as a premonitory sign of polyarteritis nodosa is probably different from the simple neuropathy and has to be included in the CIC disease. The frequency of these lesions is low, and estimated at less than 1% (Lowy 1965).

Real neuropsychiatric complications are very rare. We could observe two cases with encephalitis symptoms and EEG disturbances during the icteric period of acute hepatitis (Willems and De Groote 1966).

Viral hepatitis is found as the etiological moment in 1% of all cases of polyradiculoneuritis (Guillain-Barré disease). This disease is a rare complication of hepatitis (Leneman 1966; Niermeijer and Gips 1975; Ng et al. 1975). It has been described as occurring in the pre-icteric phase or rather later, or even during chronic hepatitis. According to most authors the prognosis is good. We describe here a case of recurrent polyradiculitis which exacerbated on several occasions during withdrawal of immunosuppression. The C_1Q binding was elelvated and an immune complex disease is suggested.

Case C. 54 years. This patient was a volonteer blood donor until in 1978 HBsAg was detected. At that moment he had no complaints and liver tests were normal.

In May 1982 he began to complain of a decrease in strength which was so marked that he could hardly walk. At the same time the values of his liver tests became more elevated. The diagnosis of polyradiculoneuritis was made. His liver test values became abnormal at that moment. Auto-antibodies were negative, no abnormal proteins were present, HBsAg, HBeAg and anti-HBc were postitive. The administration of methylprednisolone (40 mg/d) was started immediately. The C_1Q binding activity was normal, but was measured after the initiation of the corticosteroid therapy.

The clinical state of the patient improved rapidly. Corticosteroids were withdrawn in July and soon after an exacerbation of the polyradiculoneuritis was noted. With readministration of the steroids the symptoms decreased again rapidly. During the following months a flare-up was noted when the therapy was dropped under 12 mg/d. At that time his C_1Q binding capacity was much elevated. Azathioprine was added to the therapy and the dose of methylprednisolone could be decreased to 4 mg/d during the following months without reappearance of the symptoms. The therapy has remained identical until the present. His general condition remains excellent. The C_1Q binding is actually within the normal limits.

Laboratory Findings.

	1982	1983	1984	1985	Nl
– GOT	21	79	44	56	$< 19U/l$
– GPT	89	235	67	77	$< 24U/l$
– HBsAg	+	+	+	+	–
– HBcAb	+	+	+	+	neg
– HBsAb	neg	neg	neg	neg	neg
– HBeAg	+	+	+	+	neg
– HBeAb	neg	neg	neg	neg	neg
– HAAb	neg	–	neg	–	neg
– γ-Glob	1.6	–	1.79	1.80	$<$ 1.5g/dl
– Autoantibodies	neg	neg	neg	neg	neg
– C_1Q binding	118	–	481	119	100%
– Abnormal proteins	neg	neg	neg	neg	neg

Blood Disturbances. Blood disturbances are either benign or extremely severe. Fortunately the last eventuality occurs only rarely.

The most common blood disturbances are the same as those seen in other viral diseases: initial leucopenia with a subsequent lymphocytosis and sometimes eosinophilia. Hemolytic anemia produced by antibodies is exceptional (Chivrac et al. 1976).

Bone marrow aplasia is the most dreaded non-liver complication in acute hepatitis. Several forms of partial aplasia have been described: namely a drop of erythrocytes, acute agranulocytosis, and thrombocytopenia (Hagler et al. 1975). A transient form of red blood cell aplasia in association with viral hepatitis occurring 4 years apart in siblings has been described (Sears et al. 1975). Severe and complete aplasia is mostly seen in HBV-negative hepatitis and is much rarer in the HBV-positive cases. It is usually a rather late phenomenon, starting in the third month after the appearance of the jaundice. However, Casciato and co-workers (1978) observed patients with aplasia as early as in the pre-icteric phase. The prognosis is extremely bad. A mortality of 90% is the rule. Bone marrow transplantation has been used with some success, others have tried testosterone therapy. The mechanism of the aplasia is unknown. It has been ascribed to auto-immune disturbance, but the final proof is lacking.

4 Chronic Hepatitis

The clinical aspects of chronic hepatitis are as variable as atypical. Many cases have a very long, even active, evolution without symptoms. Most of these patients are chance findings. Other patients complain of an intense fatigue sometimes accompanied by a loss of appetite and vague discomfort in the right hypochondrium. In other cases and mostly in the very active group, the symptoms of acute hepatitis may be observed. We will not discuss these because they are well known. It must be stressed that there is only a poor correlation between symptoms and severity. Table 1 gives the clinical features in a series of 65 consecutive patients.

The very important question concerning chronic hepatitis is the frequency of evolution of the acute disease into a chronic one. The figures from the literature are certainly somewhat erratic and need comment and further study. One fact remains unshaken until now: hepatitis A does not become chronic. In some cases it may last longer than usual: duration of more than 6 months was observed by us. Even when a rather late biopsy of acute HAV hepatitis shows features of chronicity, such as piecemeal necrosis, the disease does not become chronic, contrary to the HBV and NANB cases (Vanstapel et al. 1983).

According to the literature, in about 5—7% of patients, acute hepatitis evolves into chronic persistent hepatitis. This figure seems rather high, and in well-controlled studies a percentage around 1% was observed. Personal uncontrolled experience favours this lowest figure. For chronic aggressive hepatitis, a percentage between 3 and 5% has been put forward. The lowest figures of about 2.5% were obtained by overall controlled studies.

Figures are available from a number of computed studies on HBsAg carriers with few symptoms or even asymptomatic. The vast majority (96%) with normal transaminases, and even 75% of those with an elevated level, had either a normal liver or chronic persistent hepatitis. In the remaining 25% with elevated transaminases more active chronic hepatitis is observed.

Table 1. Clinical features in 65 consecutive patients with mild chronic active hepatitis observed at the University Hospital Gasthuisberg, Leuven

	N	%		N	%
Liver:			Fatigue	23	35
Painful	25	38	Pain R hipochondr.	22	34
Enlarged	43	66	Anorexia	13	20
Spleen:			Fat intolerance	10	15
Enlarged	19	20	Pruritus	4	6
Jaundice:	16	24			

In NANB patients, the evolution toward chronicity seems more frequent. In the post-transfusion cases the figures vary between 20 and 50%, many authors find percentages near 50%. The incidence in sporadic cases is less, and amounts to ca. 10–20%. The cause of this difference is not known.

The prognosis of chronic hepatitis is very variable, and is difficult to predict although certain trends may be distinguished. The majority of CPH patients have an excellent long-term evolution. Some authors claim that this disease never progresses into cirrhosis (Becker et al. 1970). However, others observe about 10% cirrhosis after a very long-term evolution (Dietrichson 1975). An exception must also be made for chronic persistent hepatitis occurring after corticosteroid treatment, which is certainly less stable and can flare up at any moment after the withdrawal of therapy.

In order to discuss prognosis, cases of chronic active hepatitis should be divided in to the mild and the more active form. We followed 54 patients with the mild form for more than 10 years. During this period half of the HBV patients became cirrhotic, as compared to 30% in the HBV-negative, presumably NANB, group. This evolution was not related to the number of exacerbations during the course of the disease. The mortality of the HBV-positive patients was significantly higher than the negative ones: 7 against 2 respectively. In the HBV+ group 4 patients out of 34 (12%) died from hepatocellular carcinoma.

The prognosis of the more active chronic hepatitis is much debated. If not treated, all patients develop cirrhosis within 1 year and half of them die within 3 years. When immunosuppressive therapy is administered, the whole outlook is changed. The evolution toward cirrhosis is slowed down or even blocked, and the prognosis become much brighter.

Of course complete eradication of the disease is only possible by universal vaccination against the HBV disease, which is already theoretically possible, and the NANB disease, when the antigen is known and the vaccine available. Furthermore, much research should be devoted to the auto-immune disease in order to reverse the ominous course of events completely.

References

Apstein MD, Koff RS (1979) Neuropsychological dysfunction in acute viral hepatitis. Digestion 19: 349–358

Bacon PA, Doherty SM, Zuckerman AJ (1975) Hepatitis-B antigen in polymyalgia rheumatica. Lancet ii: 476–478

Baxter JH, Asworth CT (1946) Renal lesions in portal cirrhosis. Arch Pathol 41: 476–488

Becker MO, Sheuer PJ, Baptista A, Sherlock S (1970) Prognosis of chronic persistent hepatitis. Lancet i: 53–57

Benhamou JP (1979) Manifestations cliniques des hépatites virales aiguës. L'hépatite virale. Masson, Paris, pp 63–82

Berger J, Hinglais N (1968) Les dépots intercapillaires d'IgA-IgG. J Urol Néphrol 74: 694–695

Brzosko W, Krawczynski K, Nazarewicz T, Morzycka M, Nowoslawski A (1974) Glomerulonephritis associated with hepatitis-B surface antigen immune complexes in children. Lancet ii: 477–481

Casciato DA, Klein CA, Kaplowitz N, Scott JL (1978) Aplastic anemia associated with type B viral hepatitis. Arch Intern Med 138: 1557–1558

Chivrac D, Capron JP, Lorriaux A (1976) Les manifestations hématologiques de l'hépatite virale aiguë commune. Arch Fr Mal Appar Dig 65: 239–248

Claudy AL, Ortonne JP, Trep C, Brugnon B (1977) Acrodermatitite papuleuse de l'adulte. A propos de 3 cas. Ann Dermatol Venereol 104: 190–194

Cochrane CG, Hawkins D (1968) Studies on circulating immune complexes II Factors governing the ability of circulating complexes to localize in blood vessels. J Exp Med 127: 137–154

Colombo M, Gerber MA, Vernace SJ, Gianotti F, Paronetto F (1977) Immune response to hepatitis B virus in children with papular acrodermatitis. Gastroenterology 73: 1103–1106

Combes B, Stastny P, Shorrey J, Eigenbrodt EH, Banera A, Hull AR, Cortes NW (1971) Glomerulonephritis with deposition of Australia antigen-antibody complexes in glomerular basement membrane. Lancet ii: 234–237

Conrad ME, Schwartz FD, Young AA (1964) Infectious hepatitis–A generalized disease. A study of renal, gastrointestinal and hematologic abnormalities. Am J Med 37: 789–801

Cosgriff TM, Arnold WJ (1977) Digital vasospasm and infarction associated with hepatitis B antigenemia. J Am Med Assoc 235: 1362–1363

Davison AM, Williams IR, Mawdsley C, Robson JS (1972) Neuropathy associated with hepatitis in patients maintained on hemodialysis. Br Med J i: 409–411

De Groote J, Fevery J, Desmet V, Van Damme B, Ray MB (1982) Kidney pathology in cirrhotic patients. In: Fiaccadori F (ed) Liver and Kidney. Physiopathological and clinical relationship. Piccin Medical Books, Padova, pp 15–23

Dietrichson O (1975) Chronic persistent hepatitis. Scand J Gastroenterol 10: 249–255

Di Matteo J, Picard R, Thibault P, Audoin J (1964) Péricardite aiguë et hépatite virale. Bull Mém Soc Méd Paris 115: 959–969

Dixon FJ, Vazques JJ, Weighe WO (1958) Pathology of serum sickness. Arch Pathol 65: 18–28

Drueke T, Barbonel C, Jungers P, Digeon M, Poisson M, Brivet F, Trecan G, Feldmann G, Crosnier J, Bach JF (1980) Hepatitis B antigen associated periarteritis nodosa in patients undergoing long-term hemodialysis. Am J Med 68: 86–90

Duffy J, Lidsky MD, Sharp JT, Davis JS, Person DA, Hollinger FB, Min KW (1976) Polyarthritis, polyarteritis and hepatitis B. Medicine 55: 19–37

Fernandez R, McCarty DJ (1971) The arthritis of viral hepatitis. Ann Intern Med 74: 207–211

Fye KH, Becker MJ, Theofilopoulos AN, Moutsopoulos H, Feldman JL, Talal N (1977) Immune complexes in hepatitis B antigen-associated periarteritis nodosa. Detection by antibody-dependent cell-mediated cytotoxicity and the Raji cell assay. Am J Med 62: 783–791

Gianotti F (1973) Papular acrodermatitis of childhood: an Australian antigen disease. Arch Dis Child 48: 794–799

Gianotti F (1978) HBsAg and papular acrodermatitis of childhood. N Engl J Med 298: 460

Gocke DJ, Hsu K, Morgan C, Bombardieri S, Lockshin M, Christian CL (1970) Polyarteritis and the Australia antigen: new association. Lancet ii: 1149–1153

Gross PA, Gerding DN (1971) Pleural effusion associated with viral hepatitis. Gastroenterology 60: 898–902

Gyorkey F, Hollinger FB, Eknogan G, Mirkovic R, Drusman GR, Gyorkey P, Vass WR, Melnick JL (1975) Immune complex glomerulonephritis, intranuclear particles in hepatocytes and in vivo clearance rates in subhuman primates inoculated with HBsAg containing plasma. Exp Mol Pathol 22: 350–365

Hagler L, Pastore RA, Bergin JJ, Wrensch MR (1975) Aplastic anaemia following viral hepatitis: report of two fatal cases and literature review. Medicine 54: 139–164

Johnson WD, Silva IC, Rocha H (1975) Serum creatine-phosphokinase in leptospirosis. J Am Med Assoc 233: 981–982

Jongedijk-Brondsted H, Stolz E, Vuzevski VD (1980) Urticaria als eerste symptoom van hepatitis-B virusinfectie. Ned Tijdschr Geneeskd 124: 971–973

Khuroo MS, Teli MR, Skidmore S, Sofi MA, Khuroo MI (1981) Incidence and severity of viral hepatitis in pregnancy. Am J Med 70: 252–255

Knecht GL, Chisari FV (1978) Reversibility of hepatitis B virus-induced glomerulonephritis and chronic active hepatitis after spontaneous clearance of serum hepatitis B surface antigen. Gastroenterology 75: 1152–1156

Knieser MR, Jenis EH, Lowental DT, Bancroft WH, Burns W, Shalhoub R (1974) Pathogenesis of renal disease associated with viral hepatitis. Arch Pathol 97: 193–200

Krikler DM (1971) Hepatitis and activity. Postgrad Med J 47: 490–492

Laverdant C, Durier R, Lemoine E (1965) Les débuts atypiques de l'hépatite virale. Revue de 21 observations émanants d'un groupement épidémique de 2876 cas. Rev Int Hépatol 15: 1199–1214

Leneman E (1966) The Gullain Barré syndrome. Definition, etiology and review of 1100 cases. Arch Intern Med 118: 139–144

Levo Y, Gorevic PD, Kassab H, Zucker-Franklin D, Gigli I, Franklin EC (1977) Mixed cryoglobulinemia–an immune complex disease often associated with hepatitis-B virus infection. Trans Assoc Am Physicians 90: 167–173

Lowy F (1965) The neuro-psychiatric complications of viral hepatitis. Can Med Assoc J 92: 237–239

McIntosh RM, Koss MN, Gocke KJ (1976) The nature and incidence of cryoproteins in hepatitis B antigen (HBsAg) positive patients. Q J Med 45: 23–38

Michas AA, Kirby JD, Kent SP (1975) Hepatitis B antigen and polymyositis. J Am Med Assoc 239: 221–222

Mowrey FH, Lundberg EA (1954) The clinical manifestations of essential polyangiitis (periarteritis nodosa) with emphasis on the hepatic manifestations. Ann Intern Med 40: 1145–1146

Neefe JR, Stokes J, Reinhold JG, Lukens FDW (1944) Hepatitis due to the injection of homologous blood products in human volunteers. J Clin Invest 23: 836–855

Ng PL, Powell LW, Campbell CB (1975) Guillain Barré syndrome during the pre-icteric phase of acute hepatitis B viral hepatitis. Aust N Z J Med 5: 367–369

Niermeijer P, Gips CH (1975) Gullain-Barré syndrome in acute HBsAg positive hepatitis. Br Med J ii: 732–733

Onion DK, Crumpacker CS, Gilliland BC (1971) Arthritis of hepatitis associated with Australian antigen. Ann Intern Med 75: 29–33

Owen RL, Shapiro H (1974) Pleural effusion, rash and energy in icteric hepatitis. N Engl J Med 291: 963–965

Patek AJ, Seegal D, Bevans M (1951) The co-existence of cirrhosis of the liver and glomerulonephritis: report of 14 cases. Am J Med Sci 221: 77–85

Popp JW, Dienstag JL, Wands JR, Block KJ (1980) Essential mixed cryoglobulinemia without evidence for hepatitis B virus infection. Ann Intern Med 92: 379–383

Ray MB (1979) Hepatitis B virus antigens in tissues. MTP Press, Lancaster

Schumacher HR, Gall EP (1974) Arthritis in acute hepatitis and chronic active hepatitis. Pathology of the synovial membrane with evidence for the presence of Australia antigen in synovial membranes. Am J Med 57: 655–664

Sears DA, George JN, Gold MS (1975) Transient red blood cell aplasia in association with viral hepatitis. Occurrence four years apart in siblings. Arch Intern Med 135: 1585–1589

Sergent JS, Lockshin MD, Christion CL, Gocke DJ (1976) Vasculitis with hepatitis B antigenemia: Long-term observations in nine patients. Medicine 55: 1–18

Soulier JP, Courouce AM, Frosner CG (1978) Anticorps anti-hépatite A dans la population française et dans les immunoglobulines plasmatiques polyvalentes des centres de transfusion (Gamma TS). Sem Hôp Paris 54: 481–488

Stevens DP, Walker J, Crum E, Roth HP, Moqkowitz RW (1972) Anicteric hepatitis presenting as polyarthritis. J Am Med Assoc 220: 687–689

Stewart JS, Farrow LJ, Clifford RE e.a. (1978) A three-year survey of viral hepatitis in West London. Q J Med 47: 365–384

Trepo C, Thivolet J (1970) Antigène Australia, hépatite virale et périartérite noueuse. Nouv Presse Méd 78: 1575

Van Damme BJCP (1977) Studies of mechanism of deposition of immune complexes in experimental glomerulonephritis. Arscia, Brussels

Vanstapel MJ, Van Steenbergen W, De Wolf-Peeters C, Desmyter J, Fevery J, De Groote J, Desmet VJ (1983) Prognostic significance of piecemeal necrosis in acute viral hepatitis. Liver 3: 46–57

Wands JR, Alpert E, Isselbacher KI (1975) Arthritis associated with chronic active hepatitis: complement activation and characterization of circulating immune complexes. Gastroenterology 19: 1286–1291

Weiss TD, Tsai CC, Baldassarre AR, Zuckner J (1978) Skin lesions in viral hepatitis. Histologic and immunofluorescent findings. Am J Med 64: 269–273

Wilkinson SP, Darres MH, Portmann R, Williams R (1978) Renal failure in otherwise uncomplicated acute viral hepatitis. Br Med J ii: 318–341

Willems J, De Groote J (1966) Neuro-psychiatrische verwikkelingen bij virus hepatitis: beschrijving van twee gevallen. Tijdschr Gastro-Enterol 9: 279–290

Hepatitis Delta Virus (HDV): Infection and Disease

P. FARCI and M. RIZZETTO[1]

1 The Virus

First described in Italian patients with chronic hepatitis B virus (HBV) infection (Rizetto et al. 1977), the delta antigen was initially considered a variant of HBV. Characterization studies in chimpanzees have instead shown that it is the internal component of a new and unique hepatitis agent, which has peculiar biological features, and requires the assistance of HBV to replicate (Rizzetto et al. 1980a). The delta agent has been recently renamed hepatitis delta virus (HDV), the internal antigen (HD-Ag) and the antibody evoked in infected hosts anti-HD (Jacobson and Dienstag 1984). The clinical significance of the new pathogen is now evident on a global scale; the HDV represents an important etiologic agent responsible for severe forms of hepatitis (Rizzetto 1983).

The virus is a 35–37 nm round particle with heterogeneous morphology. It is coated with HBsAg provided by the host HBV infection, but contains a specific protein, the HD-Ag, and a small RNA genome (Rizzetto et al. 1980b); the virion is disrupted by several physicochemical treatments without releasing a nucleocapsid (Bonino et al. 1984). The HD-Ag, the only identified antigenic expression of the new pathogen, is a protein of molecular weight of approximately 68,000 (Rizzetto et al. 1980c). The genome is a linear RNA of 1.75 kilobases, unrelated to HBV-DNA and to host ribosomal or other RNA viruses (Hoyer et al. 1983). Using the recombinant DNA technology, the HDV-RNA has been cloned and partially sequenced. A sensitive cDNA probe is now available for the identification of HDV-RNA in serum by blot hybridization (Denniston et al. 1984).

As a defective virus depending on HBsAg synthesis for its replication, the host range of the HDV extends to the primate species susceptible to HBV infection (Rizzetto 1985). It can also be transmitted to the woodchuck, a rodent susceptible to infection with the woodchuck strain of Hepadna viruses, a family of viruses antigenically and genetically distinct from HBV that share with it a common morphology and genome structure; interestingly, the virion particles isolated from the blood of woodchucks have shown the same hybrid composition as those observed in primates (Ponzetto et al. 1984). Electron and immune electron microscopy studies performed in human and chimpanzee liver positive for HD-Ag have failed to identify ultrastructural morphologies suggestive of virus-like particles specific to HDV infection (Canese et al. 1979; 1984; Kamimura et al. 1983).

---

1   Clinica Medica I, University of Cagliari, Italy, Division of Gastroenterology, Molinette, Torino, Italy

Viral Hepatitis, ed. by F. Callea et al.
© Springer-Verlag Berlin Heidelberg 1986

2 Modes of Infection

In view of the obligatory link of the HDV with the HBV, HDV infection occurs in the presence of concomitant HBV infection. The modes of infection are simultaneous co-infection with HBV or superinfection of a HBsAg carrier. Persons with anti-HBs, being immune to HBV infection, are not susceptible to HDV. It is therefore likely that the outcome of HDV is essentially determined by the course and outcome of the underlying HBV infection. Coinfection usually leads to an acute self-limited hepatitis, which cannot be distinguished clinically from hepatitis B. Since the HBs antigenemia necessary to support HDV is transient, the pathogenic effect of HBV is limited and the outcome is usually complete recovery, as typical of acute type B hepatitis; coinfected individuals are not at higher risk of chronic HDV hepatitis than those acutely infected with HBV alone (Smedile et al. 1981). Coinfection, however, is a cause of severe or fulminant hepatitis (Smedile et al. 1982a) or of a biphasic hepatitis with two amino-transferase peaks corresponding to the HBV and HDV events.

Different clinical and serological features develop when HDV infects individuals who carry the HBsAg (Smedile et al. 1981), as the pre-existing HB viremia provides the biological background for the full expression of the virulence of HDV. The clinical outcome is variable; it may be an acute, often severe hepatitis (De Cock et al. 1984), appearing as an exacerbation of pre-existing HBV disease or as a new hepatitis in asymptomatic HBsAg carriers. If the HBsAg state is unknown, the acute hepatitis may be misdiagnosed as classical acute hepatitis B. The correct diagnosis is suggested by a negative test for IgM anti-core and confirmed by positive HDV serology (Farci et al. 1983). In the sick carrier, the HDV superinfection aggravates the underlying HBV disease and portends liver failure (Raimondo et al. 1983). As the HBsAg state represents also the sole terrain permitting the maintenance of HDV replication, carriers superinfected by HDV are at high risk of developing a progressive hepatitis.

A minority of superinfected carriers experience a self-limited hepatitis and clear the virus (Smedile et al. 1981); in one patient the HBsAg state was terminated coincidentally with the acute infection (Moenstrup et al. 1983).

3 Diagnosis

The virus is identified by the presence of HD-Ag. The infection evokes an antibody response of IgM and of IgG class, which is thus an indirect indicator of exposure to HDV.

The HD-Ag may be detected in the serum and in the liver (Crivelli et al. 1983a). In serum it can be measured by radio- and enzyme-linked immunoassay (Rizzetto et al. 1980c; Crivelli et al. 1981). Its detection requires the addition of detergents to disrupt the virion and expose the antigen. In liver, HD-Ag is demonstrated in unfixed and fixed tissue, by immunofluorescence and immunoperoxidase techniques (Recchia et al. 1981). The localization is nuclear and rarely cytoplasmic.

Total anti-HD, which measures predominantly antibody of IgG class, is determined by solid-phase radio and enzyme-linked immunoassay, using HD-Ag from primate or rodent liver (Rizzetto et al. 1980c). An Elisa has been developed using HD-Ag obtained from serum of patients with acute HDV hepatitis (Shattock and Morgan 1984). The radioimmunoassay for IgM anti-HD is based on the capture of IgM in the serum test by an anti-human μ attached to a solid phase (Smedile et al. 1982b) with the subsequent addition of HD-Ag and demonstration of the IgM anti-HD–HD-Ag binding with labeled IgG anti-HD.

Though the HD-Ag can be occasionally detected in serum of acute HDV infection, diagnosis of acute hepatitis D is most frequently made by a positive test for IgM anti-HD (Smedile et al. 1982b). This is because the HD-Ag is expressed for a short time during the acute infection and the immune response is usually a transient appearance of IgM anti-HD not followed by secondary conversion to the homologous IgG antibody. HD-antigenemia, however, seems to correlate with the degree of liver damage and the finding of this marker points therefore to a severe illness. The immune response is more prominent following HDV superinfection of a HBsAg carrier. There is more often a phase of early HD-antigenemia coincident with intra-hepatic production of antigen, followed by seroconversion to IgM anti-HD and then to a IgG reaction.

The diagnosis of chronic HDV infection is established by the detection of intra-hepatic HD-Ag and by the persisitence of high titered anti-HD in serum. Despite the production of HD-Ag in the liver, HD-antigenemia cannot be shown by conventional immunoassay during the chronic phase (Rizzetto 1983). Chronic HDV infection seems associated with continuing synthesis of IgM anti-HD (Smedile et al. 1982b), and testing for IgM anti-HD helps to discriminate between current and past HDV infection. The IgM test also provides prognostic information on the course of chronic HDV hepatitis (Farci et al. 1986). Testing for HDV-RNA adds another parameter to the diagnosis; the finding of the genome correlates with the presence of intrahepatic HD-Ag and serum IgM anti-HD (Smedile et al. 1984).

4 Clinical Aspects

The HDV appears to be highly pathogenic, as hepatitis has occurred in all the animals experimentally infected with this virus (Rizzetto et al. 1980a) and a progressive shortening of the incubation period with an increase in the severity of the hepatitis was seen in sequential HDV infections (Gerin et al. 1982); the acute hepatitis seen in chimpanzees superinfected by the HDV was indeed the most severe disease observed during studies of experimental viral hepatitis (Purcell et al. 1983).

In man, the clinical syndromes and the outcome of HDV infection are variable. Three responses to the infection have been observed, acute hepatitis, chronic hepatitis, subclinical hepatitis.

Coinfection of HDV with HBV results usually in hepatitis resembling infection with the hepatitis B virus alone (Smedile et al. 1981). The patients are not prone to develop chronic disease, recovery is the rule but the double viral infection may induce a fulminant hepatitis (Rizzetto 1983). Evidence of primary HDV infection has been found in up to 60% of the patients from different series of fulminant HBsAg hepatitis (Smedile et al. 1982). Serological analysis of these individuals, however, has also shown that a high proportion lacked the IgM antibody to HBcAg, suggesting that another mechanism responsible for the severe disease is superinfection of a HBsAg carrier. The ominous effect of HDV superinfection in carriers was documented during an outbreak of hepatitis D in Yucpa Indians in Venezuela (Hadler et al. 1984), an area where a high prevalence of HBsAg carriers was paramount in determining a fatal outcome in many patients (18%) and a high rate of chronic HDV hepatitis (68%).

Acute HDV hepatitis occurring in unknown HBV carriers may present a difficult diagnostic problem, as it can be misinterpreted as an acute type B hepatitis (Farci et al. 1983). In retrospective analysis, markers of the HDV were found in 81 and 67% of patients collected in Naples and Cagliari, whose apparent type B hepatitis became chronic.

It is likely that the majority of patients with chronic HDV hepatitis are carriers of HBV who became superinfected by the HDV.

The chronic disease caused by the HDV is often severe and progressive (Aricò et al. 1978, Colombo et al. 1983; Govindarajan et al. 1983).

One study has demonstrated that the expression of intra-hepatic HD antigen was associated with the histological diagnosis of chronic active hepatitis or cirrhosis in over 90% of cases (Rizzetto et al. 1983), and another study indicates that hepatitis type D in HBsAg carriers may very rapidly approach cirrhosis, as progression from acute disease to nodular transformation was observed in a period of less than 1 year (Saracco et al. 1986). The association of HDV with an increased level of inflammatory activity has been also confirmed in children (Farci et al. 1985b). The frequency of HDV in HBsAg-positive hepatocellular carcinoma is low (Govindarajan et al. 1984); this may relate to the rapid progression of the liver disease, which diminishes the life expectancy of the patient, so that death occurs before development of hepatocellular carcinoma.

Several clinical features are characteristic of patients with chronic HDV hepatitis. Over 50% of the patients with HDV disease report a previous episode of acute hepatitis that possibly represents the time of HDV superinfection (Rizzetto et al. 1983) and in many, autoantibodies against the microsomal membranes of the liver and kidney (Crivelli et al. 1983b), the basal cell layer of the rat forestomach (Zauli et al. 1984) and the epithelial cells of the thymus (Magnius et al. 1985) are found.

The majority of the patient with chronic HDV infection are anti-HBe-positive and HBV-DNA-negative in serum (Rizzetto et al. 1983); this was confirmed in children, who in the absence of HDV infection are usually HBeAg-positive (Farci et al. 1985a). The biological relation of HDV to the HBeAg/anti-HBe state is controversial, as one study reported no significant inhibition of HBV replication in two carriers superinfected by HDV (Farci et al. 1985b) but other studies have shown a significant depression of HBV-DNA synthesis accompanied by seroconversion from HBeAg to anti-HBe in superinfected individuals.

The histological features are nonspecific (Verme et al. 1983). An eosinophilic granulation of the cytoplasm of the hepatocytes and a marked lobular infiltration by inflammatory cells are more common in HDV than HBV liver disease. Genetic factors do not appear to be involved (Forzani et al. 1984).

Infection with the HDV may be subclinical and a cause of asymptomatic liver disease. Antibody to HDV was found in a high proportion of asymptomatic Greek carriers with histologically important chronic hepatitis (Hadzyiannis et al. 1984) and this condition was also well documented in Italy among asymptomatic blood donors: a significant proportion of those with anti-HD had biochemical or histological evidence of advanced liver disease (Aricò et al. 1985).

References

Aricò S, Rizzetto M, Crivelli O, Canese MG, Zanetti A, Ponzetto A, Ferrari G, Bonino F, Pera A, Verme G (1978) The clinical significance of a new antigen/antibody system (delta/anti-delta) in chronic carriers of the HBsAg. Ital J Gastroenterol 10: 146–151

Aricò S, Aragona M, Rizzetto M, Caredda F, Zanetti A, Marinucci G, Diana S, Farci P, Arnone M, Caporaso N, Ascione A, Dentico P, Pastore G, Raimondo G, Craxi A (1985) Clinical significance of antibody to the hepatitis delta virus in symptomless HBsAg carriers. Lancet 17: 356–358

Bonino F, Hoyer B, Shih JWK, Rizzetto M, Purcell RH, Gerin JL (1984) Delta hepatitis agent: structural and antigenic properties of the delta-associated particle. Infect Immun 43: 1000–1005

Canese MG, Rizzetto M, Aricò S, Crivelli O, Zanetti AR, Macchiorlatti E, Ponzetto A, Leone L, Mollo F, Verme G (1979) An ultrastructural and immunohistochemical study on the delta antigen associated with hepatitis B. J Pathol 128: 169–175

Canese MG, Rizzetto M, Novara R, London WT, Purcell RH (1984) Experimental infection with the HBsAg associated delta agent (δ). An ultrastructural study. J Med Virol 13: 63–72

Colombo B, Cambieri R, Rumi MG, Ronchi G, Del Ninno E, De Franchis R (1983) Long-term superinfection in HBsAg carriers and its relationship with the course of chronic hepatitis. Gastroenterology 85: 235–239

Crivelli O, Rizzetto M, Lavarini C, Smedile A, Gerin JL (1981) Enzyme-linked immunosorbent assay for detection of antibody to the HBsAg-associated delta antigen. J Clin Microbiol 14 (2): 172–177

Crivelli O, Shih JWK, Rizzetto M (1983a) Methods for detection of the delta antigen and antibody in liver and serum. In: Verme G, Bonino F, Rizzetto M (eds) Viral hepatitis and delta infection. Progress in clinical and biological research, vol 143. Liss, New York, pp 121–126

Crivelli O, Lavarini C, Chiaberge E, Amoroso A, Farci P, Negro F, Rizzetto M (1983b) Microsomal autoantibodies in chronic infection with the HBsAg-associated delta agent. Clin Exp Immunol 54: 232–238

De Cock KM, Govindarajan S, Redeker AG (1984) Fulminant delta hepatitis in chronic hepatitis B infection. J Am Med Assoc 252: 2746–2748

Denniston KJ, Wells F, Engle R, Hoyer B, Gerin JL (1984) cDNA cloning of delta agent associated RNA and preliminary nucleotide sequence determination. In: Vyas GN, Dienstag JL, Hoofnagle JA (eds) Viral hepatitis and liver disease. Abst LA 1: 696

Farci P, Smedile A, Lavarini C, Piantino P, Crivelli O, Caporaso N, Toti M, Bonino F, Rizzetto M (1983) Delta hepatitis in inapparent carriers of hepatitis B surface antigen. Gastroenterology 85: 669–673

Farci P, Aragona M, Crivelli O, Smedile A, Gerin JL, Lindsey I, Balestrieri A, Thomas HC, Rizzetto M (1986) Diagnostic and prognostic significance of the IgM antibody to the Hepatitis Delta Virus. J Am Med Assoc 255: 1443–1446

Farci P, Barbera C, Novara C, Bortolotti F, Vajro P, Caporaso N, Vegnente A, Ansaldi N, Rizzetto M, Tolentino P, Calzia R (1985a) Infection with the Delta agent in children. Gut 26: 4–7

Farci P, Karayiannis P, Jowett T, Balestrieri A, Thomas HC (1985b) The effect of acute and chronic HDV infection on HBV replication: Are anti-HBe positive HBV carriers without HBV replication more susceptible to HDV superinfection? (submitted)

Forzani B, Actis GC, Amoroso A, Borelli I, Curtoni ES, Rumi MG, Picciotto A, Marinucci G, Freni MA, Rizzetto M (1984) HLA-DR antigens in HBsAg-positive chronic active liver disease with and without associated delta infection. Hepatology 4: 1107–1110

Gerin JL, Ponzetto A, London WT, Sly DL, Purcell R (1982) Serial passage of the delta agent (δ) in chimpanzees. Fed Proc 41: 445

Govindarajan S, Kanel GC, Peters RL (1983) Prevalence of antibody among chronic Hepatitis B virus infected patients in the Los Angeles area: its correlation with liver biopsy diagnosis. Gastroenterology 85: 160–162

Govindarajan S, Hevia FJ, Peters RL (1984) Prevalence of delta antigen/antibody in B-viral-associated hepatocellular carcinoma. Cancer 53: 1962–1964

Hadler SC, De Monzon M, Ponzetto A, Anzola E, Rivero D, Mondolfi A, Bracho A, Fracis DP, Ageber M, Thung S, Gerin JL, Maynard JE, Popper M, Purcell HR (1984) An epidemic of severe hepatitis due to delta virus infection in Yupca Indians of Venezuela. Ann Intern Med 100: 339–349

Hadziyannis S, Hatzakis A, Karamanos B (1984) Clinical features of chronic delta (δ) infection. In: Vyas GN, Dienstag JL, Hoofnagle JH (eds) Viral hepatitis and liver disease. Abst SAT-LA: 18

Hoyer B, Bonino F, Ponzetto A, Denniston K, Nelson J, Purcell RH, Gerin JL (1983) Properties of delta-associated ribonucleic acid. In: Verme G, Bonino F, Rizzetto M (eds) Viral hepatitis and delta infection. Progress in clinical and biological research, vol 143. Liss, New York, pp 91–97

Jacobson IM, Dienstag JL (1984) The delta hepatitis agent: Viral hepatitis type D. Gastroenterology 86: 1614–1617

Kamimura T, Ponzetto A, Bonino F, Feinstone SM, Gerin JL, Purcell RH (1983) Cytoplasmic tubular structures in liver of HBsAg carrier chimpanzees infected with δ agent and comparison with cytoplasmic structures in non-A, non-B hepatitis. Hepatology 3: 631–637

Magnius LO, Lenkei R, Norder H, Biberfeld G, Mushahwar IK (1985) Autoantibodies ot thymic epithelial cells in hepatitis B virus associated δ infection. J Infect Dis 152: 232

Moenstrup T, Hansonn BG, Widell A, Nordenfelt E (1983) Clinical aspects of delta infection. Br Med J 286: 87–90

Ponzetto A, Cote PJ, Popper H, Hoyer BH, London WT, Ford EC, Bonino F, Purcell RH, Gerin JL (1984) Transmission of the hepatitis B virus-associated δ agent to the eastern woodchuck. Proc Natl Acad Sci USA 81: 2208–2212

Purcell RH, Gerin JL, Rizzetto M, Ponzetto A, Bonino F, London WT (1983) Experimental transmission of the delta agent to chimpanzees. In: Verme G, Bonino F, Rizzetto M (eds) Viral hepatitis and delta infection. Progress in clinical and biological research, vol 143. Liss, New York, pp 79–89

Raimondo G, Longo G, Squadrito G (1983) Exacerbation of chronic liver disease due to hepatitis B surface antigen after delta infection. Br Med J 286: 845

Recchia S, Rizzi R, Acquaviva F, Rizzetto M, Tison V, Bonino F, Verme G (1981) Immunoperoxidase staining of the HBV-associated delta antigen in paraffinated liver specimens. Pathologica 73: 773–777

Rizzetto M (1983) The delta agent. Hepatology 3: 729–737

Rizzetto M (1985) Delta hepatitis. Present status. J Hepatol 1: 187–193

Rizzetto M, Canese MG, Aricò S, Crivelli O, Trepo C, Bonino F, Verme G (1977) Immunofluorescence detection of a new antigen/antibody system (delta/anti-delta) associated with hepatitis B virus in liver and serum of HBsAg carriers. Gut 18: 997–1003

Rizzetto M, Canese MG, Gerin JL, London WT, Sly LD, Purcell RH (1980a) Transmission of hepatitis B virus-associated delta-antigen to chimpanzees. J Infect Dis 121: 590–602

Rizzetto M, Hoyer B, Canese MG, Shih JWK, Purcell RH, Gerin JL (1980b) Delta antigen: the association of delta antigen with hepatitis B surface antigen and ribonucleic acid in the serum of delta infected chimpanzees. Proc Natl Acad Sci USA 77: 6124–6128

Rizzetto M, Shih JWK, Gerin JL (1980c) The hepatitis B virus-associated delta antigen (δ). Isolation from liver, development of solid phase radioimmunoassay for delta and anti-delta and partial characterization of delta. J Immunol 125: 318–324

Rizzetto M, Verme G, Recchia S, Bonino F, Farci P, Aricò S, Calzia R, Picciotto A, Colombo M, Popper H (1983) Chronic HBsAg hepatitis with intrahepatic expression of delta antigen. An active and progressive disease unresponsive to immuno-suppressive treatment. Ann Intern Med 98: 437–441

Saracco C, Rosina F, Brunetto M, Amoroso P, Caredda F, Farci P, Piantino P, Bonino F, Rizzetto M (1986) Subacute, rapidly progressive HBsAg hepatitis in Italy: a syndrome of hepatitis delta virus superinfection (submitted)

Shattock AG, Morgan M (1984) Sensitive enzyme-immunoassay for the detection of delta antigen and anti-delta using serum as the delta antigen source. J Med Virol 13: 73–82

Smedile A, Dentico P, Zanetti A, Sagnelli E, Nordenfelt E, Actis G, Rizzetto M (1981) Infection with the HBV-associated delta (δ) agent in HBsAg carriers. Gastroenterology 81: 992–997

Smedile A, Farci P, Verme G, Caredda F, Cargnel A, Caporaso M, Dentico P, Trepo C, Opolon P, Gimson A, Vergani D, Williams R, Rizzetto M (1982a) Influence of delta infection on severity of hepatitis B. Lancet II: 945–947

Smedile A, Lavarini C, Crivelli O, Raimondo G, Fassone M, Rizzetto M (1982b) Radioimmunoassay detection of IgM antibodies to the HBV-associated delta (δ) antigen, clinical significance in δ infection. J. Med Virol 9: 131–138

Smedile A, Rizzetto M, Bonino F, Gerin JL, Hoyer B (1984) Serum Delta-associated RNA (DAR) in chronic HBV carriers infected with the delta agent. In: Vyas GN, Dienstag JL, Hoofnagle JH (eds) Viral hepatitis and liver disease. Abst 3A 9: 613

Verme G, Rocca G, Rizzi R, Mollo F, David E, Solcia E, Sessa F (1983) Histopatology of chronic delta hepatitis. In: Verme G, Bonino F, Rizzetto M (eds) Viral hepatitis and delta infection. Progress in clinical and biological research, vol 143. Liss, New York, pp 169–176

Zauli D, Fusconi M, Crespi C, Bianchi F, Craxi A, Pisi E (1984) Close association between basal cell layer antibodies (BCLA) and HBV-associated chronic delta infection. Hepatology 4: 1103–1106

The Pathology of Acute Viral Hepatitis

P.J. SCHEUER[1]

All forms of acute hepatitis have certain pathological features in common. There is inflammatory cell infiltration of acini and portal tracts, and evidence of liver-cell damage, with or without frank necrosis. The inflammatory infiltrate is mainly composed of lymphoid cells, including plasma cells (Mietkiewski and Scheuer 1985), but a few segmented leucocytes are commonly seen. Kupffer cells and portal macrophages are enlarged, and may contain diastase PAS-positive ceroid pigment with or without iron. Liver-cell damage takes the form of swelling or shrinkage. The cytoplasm of affected cells may be deeply acidophilic. Rounded acidophil (Councilman) bodies are often present. Focal or confluent areas of cell loss are marked by inflammatory cells and Kupffer cells, as well as by condensation of the reticulin framework. Another feature of liver-cell damage is the presence of cholestasis in the form of bile plugs in canaliculi. All the above parenchymal changes are often most severe near terminal hepatic venules and least severe near portal tracts, but may be found throughout the acini. In a few patients, cell damage and necrosis are predominantly periportal. Portal inflammation, with or without a periportal component, is a constant feature of acute viral hepatitis, and may be mistaken for the lesions of chronic persistent or chronic active hepatitis. Bile ducts may show epithelial irregularities or frank damage, with vacuolated, pseudostratified epithelium.

This description refers to classical acute hepatitis with spotty (focal) necrosis. Other morphological forms include acute hepatitis with bridging necrosis, hepatitis with panacinar or multiacinar necrosis, and hepatitis with periportal necrosis. Bridging necrosis linking portal tracts with terminal hepatic venules probably represents confluent necrosis of acinar zones 3. It signifies severe liver-cell damage, but is not necessarily followed by chronic hepatitis. It is important to distinguish recent bridging necrosis from fibrosis, in order to avoid overdiagnosis of chronic active hepatitis. In this respect it is helpful to examine a stain for elastic fibres (e.g. orcein), because these are abundant in chronic septa but absent from areas of recent collapse (Scheuer and Maggi 1980). Panacinar necrosis and multiacinar necrosis, involving total or near-total destruction of acinar parenchyma, is usually seen in patients with fulminant acute hepatitis clinically, but can also be found in limited areas in less severe attacks. Periportal necrosis occasionally dominates the histological picture of acute hepatitis, and, like bridging necrosis, is apt to lead to overdiagnosis of chronic active hepatitis. The distinction is best

1 Department of Histopathology, The Royal Free Hospital School of Medicine
University of London, London NW3 2QG, United Kingdom

Viral Hepatitis, ed. by F. Callea et al.
© Springer-Verlag Berlin Heidelberg 1986

made by careful assessment of the clinical circumstances and of the other parenchymal changes on liver biopsy.

These various forms of acute hepatitis can be caused by infection with hepatitis A virus (HAV), hepatitis B virus (HBV) with or without the delta agent (hepatitis D virus, HDV), or one of the non-A, non-B (NANB) viruses. There is considerable overlap between the histological features of these infections, and no absolute criteria exist for their histological differentiation. Nevertheless, certain features and patterns have become evident. In type A hepatitis, a cholestatic course is common clinically, and correspondingly cholestasis is often seen histologically, sometimes with little accompanying necrosis or acinar inflammation (Teixeira et al. 1982). Periportal hepatitis is also common, and may either be seen on its own or combined with cholestasis (Teixeira et al. 1982; Abe et al. 1982). The portal and periportal infiltrate is characteristically rich in plasma cells. Intense portal inflammation is also seen in marmosets infected with HAV, together with liver-cell swelling and cholestasis (Karayiannis et al. 1986). Liver-cell damage is more striking, and inflammatory infiltration less, after pretreatment with corticosteroids, consistent with a possible (but unproven) cytopathic component; on the other hand, virus antigen can be demonstrated before the onset of hepatitis, and the latter corresponds with the appearance of antibody, indicating that immunological factors probably play an important part in the pathogenesis of the liver lesion. Type B hepatitis is often characterized by severe necrosis, and by close contact between hepatocytes and lymphocytes. The surface antigen, HBsAg, is only rarely demonstrable in liver tissue during the acute attack and HBsAg-rich ground-glass hepatocytes are only found in chronic disease. Diagnosis therefore rests on serological rather than histological information. Infection with HBV may be complicated by coinfection or superinfection with HDV, which may lead to severe chronic disease or to fulminant acute hepatitis (Smedile et al. 1982). The delta antigen can be demonstrated by immunoperoxidase in formalin-fixed, paraffin-embedded tissue. HDV infection is characterized histologically by substantial inflammation and necrosis.

NANB hepatitis has proved difficult to delineate accurately because of the current lack of widely applicable and reproducible serum markers. A number of histological features and patterns have been described. In series of biopsies from patients with short-incubation NANB hepatitis following factor VIII infusion, lymphocytic infiltration of sinusoids was the dominant feature (Bamber et al. 1981). There may be substantial fatty change, and bile duct damage associated with the formation of lymphoid follicles in portal tracts (Schmid et al. 1982). Acidophilic degeneration of hepatocytes and the formation of many acidophil bodies have been noted. A common feature of NANB virus infections is the presence of acinar (lobular) necrosis even in chronic forms (Dienes et al. 1982). This may lead to confusion between chronic and acute disease histologically. Several types of nuclear particle and cytoplasmic structure have been found in NANB hepatitis by electron microscopy, but are not currently thought to offer a specific diagnostic criterion (De Vos et al. 1983).

Finally, infection with more than one hepatitis is now known to be common, especially in patients whose lifestyle or special risk factors (e.g. haemophilia) lead to multiple exposure. This presents both clinician and pathologist with a diagnostic challenge.

References

Abe H, Beninger PR, Ikejiri M, Setoyama H, Sata M, Tanikawa K (1982) Light microscopic findings of liver biopsy specimens from patients with hepatitis type A and comparison with type B. Gastroenterology 82: 938–947

Bamber M, Murray A, Arborgh BAM, Scheuer PJ, Kernoff PB, Thomas HC, Sherlock S (1981) Short incubation non-A, non-B hepatitis transmitted by factor VIII concentrates in patients with congenital coagulation disorders. Gut 22: 854–859

Dienes HP, Popper H, Arnold W, Lobeck H (1982) Histologic observations in human hepatitis non-A, non-B. Hepatology 2: 562–571

De Vos R, Vanstapel MJ, Desmyter J, De Wolf-Peeters C, De Groote G, Colaert J, Mortelmans J, De Groote J, Fevery J, Desmet V (1983) Are nuclear particles specific for non-A, non-B hepatitis? Hepatology 3: 532–544

Karayiannis P, Jowett T, Enticott M , Moore D, Pignatelli M, Brenes F, Scheuer PJ, Thomas HC (1986) Hepatitis A virus (HAV) replication in tamarins and host immune response in relation to pathogenesis of liver cell damage in acute HAV infection. J Med Virol 18: 261–276

Mietkiewski JM, Scheuer PJ (1985) Immunoglobulin-containing plasma cells in acute hepatitis. Liver 5: 84–88

Scheuer PJ, Maggi G (1980) Hepatic fibrosis and collapse: histological distinction by orcein staining. Histopathology 4: 487–490

Schmid M, Pirovino M, Altorfer J, Gudat F, Bianchi L (1982) Acute hepatitis non-A, non-B; are there any specific light microscopic features? Liver 2: 61–67

Smedile A, Farci P, Verme G, Caredda F, Cargnel A, Caporaso N, Dentico P, Trepo C, Opolon P, Gimson A, Vergani D, Williams R, Rizzetto M (1982) Influence of delta infection on severity of hepatitis B. Lancet ii: 945–947

Teixeira MR Jr, Weller IVD, Murray A, Bamber M, Thomas HC, Sherlock S, Scheuer PJ (1982) The pathology of hepatitis A in man. Liver 2: 53–60

Histopathology of Chronic Viral Hepatitis

V.J. DESMET[1]

1 Introduction

The histopathological changes observed in the liver biopsy in chronic hepatitis are extremely variable, due to variations in etiology, course of disease, disease activity, and evolutionary stage.

For therapeutic purposes, etiology and disease activity are the most important considerations. Histopathological classification of chronic viral hepatitis is mainly based on disease activity, delineating milder and more severe categories.

Since 1968, chronic hepatitis has been subdivided into chronic persistent (CPH) and chronic active (or aggressive) (CAH) hepatitis (De Groote et al. 1968). The usefulness of this subdivision is reflected in the observation that the histopathological features of CPH are usually associated with a favorable prognosis (Chadwick et al. 1979), whereas CAH has a serious tendency to develop into cirrhosis (De Groote et al. 1978).

This simple classification is, of course, not entirely satisfactory (Degott and Potet 1983). One reason is that the concept "chronic hepatitis" covers a broad spectrum of liver alterations, ranging from near-normal liver histology to severe lesions including necrosis, inflammation, fibrosis, and architectural disturbance (cirrhosis); the original classification drew its borderlines mainly on the basis of inflammatory changes, with less emphasis on necrotizing lesions. A second, and more important danger is that the subdivision in CPH and CAH has been misunderstood by some to distinguish two different disease entities, whereas they intend to delineate two broad categories of disease activity. A third problem is that subdivision of a broad spectrum into two groups does not specify the broad range of variants within each group.

A fourth handicap of any subdivision in a broad spectrum disease lies in the fact that it draws somewhat arbitrary borderlines in what, in fact, corresponds to a continuum, so that "borderline cases" always remain a problem.

Several studies during the last decade have emphasized particular features, resulting in a more complex categorization of chronic inflammatory liver disease. Distinction is still made between a group of mild ("persistent") variants and a group of more severe ("active" or "aggressive") variants of chronic hepatitis.

---

1 Universitair Ziekenhuis Sint Rafael Laboratorium voor Histochemie en Cytochemie
Katholieke Universiteit Leuven, 3000 Leuven, Belgium

Viral Hepatitis, ed. by F. Callea et al.
© Springer-Verlag Berlin Heidelberg 1986

2 Milder Variants of Chronic Viral Hepatitis

Chronic Persistent Hepatitis (CPH). This variant represents the originally defined type of CPH, and morphologically corresponds to "portal" hepatitis (Popper and Schaffner 1971).

Portal tracts are infiltrated by mononuclear cells comprising mainly lymphocytes. In typical CPH, the inflammatory cells are restricted within the limits of the portal connective tissue: there is no piecemeal necrosis.

Cases presenting minimal degrees of periportal extension of the inflammatory cells can be considered as "borderline" with CAH, and represent, strictly speaking, a minimal degree of CAH (Lenoir et al. 1978). Lobular architecture is preserved and parenchymal damage is minimal.

In chronic persistent hepatitis due to hepatitis B virus (HBV) a large number of ground-glass hepatocytes (GGH) (Hadziyannis 1981) may be observed.

This histological picture of "portal hepatitis" is not specific for CPH, but represents only one of the many causes of portal inflammation. Differential diagnosis includes, for example, late residual of declining acute hepatitis, nonspecific reactive hepatitis, and primary biliary cirrhosis (Scheuer 1977; Bianchi 1983).

It is important to realize that nonrepresentative biopsies in CAH may only comprise portal tracts with "portal hepatitis" devoid of piecemeal necrosis, so that the disease activity is underestimated as CPH. Therefore, a histopathological picture of "portal hepatitis" should only be interpreted as CPH after consideration of the clinical and biochemical features (Thaler 1974).

Chronic Lobular Hepatitis (CLH). This term was introduced in 1971 (Popper and Schaffner) to describe a lobular lesion of necrosis and inflammation as seen in classical acute hepatitis, but on a chronic time scale.

Piecemeal necrosis and confluent necrosis (see below) are not part of the picture of CLH.

Since the histological picture is that of acute hepatitis, the diagnosis of CLH can only be made after consideration of the clinical history of the patient. CLH may be caused by HBV and by non-A, non-B hepatitis virus, and carries in general a good prognosis (Liaw et al. 1982).

Chronic Hepatitis with Nonspecific Histological Changes. Nonspecific Reactive Hepatitis (NSRH). Recent studies in the Far East (Liaw et al. 1984) have drawn attention to the observation that a subgroup of patients with chronic hepatitis, in spite of otherwise great similarity with CPH, have fluctuating courses with remarkable biochemical changes and histological features of CLH and even CAH.

This subgroup of NSRH is characterized by low-grade or minimal changes, such as occasional foci of necrosis, mobilization and increase of Kupffer cells, and mild portal inflammation, usually in only some portal tracts. In short, in NSRH the lobular lesions are milder than in CLH and the portal inflammation is milder than in CPH (Liaw et al. 1984; Popper and Schaffner 1976). It was concluded that NSRH should be classified as a variant independent of CPH, apparently corresponding to a remission phase of CLH, which itself corresponds to a relapse phase (Liaw et al. 1984).

Chronic Septal Hepatitis (CSH). Chronic septal hepatitis (Gerber and Vernace 1974) can be considered as a remission phase of chronic active hepatitis, during which the disease activity has regressed to the lower level of CPH.

In such cases the inflammatory infiltration is comparable to that of CPH: restricted within the portal connective tissue without intraparenchymal extension or piecemeal necrosis. There is, however, increased fibrosis in the form of periportal connective tissue septa, which are thought to represent the burnt-out scars of previously more active inflammation. In spite of the septa, there is no nodular remodeling of the parenchyma and no cirrhosis. The prognosis of CSH is not as good as that of simple CPH.

3 More Severe Variants of Chronic Viral Hepatitis

Variants of chronic hepatitis with a more severe degree of activity are termed chronic active or aggressive hepatitis. The histopathological hallmark of this more serious group of conditions is piecemeal necrosis. This lesion may be present in mild or extensive degree, reflecting different levels of disease activity.

However, piecemeal necrosis is not the only variable indicating severity of disease. Lobular parenchymal lesions also occur to a variable extent, ranging from mild focal necrosis to widespread multilobular necrosis, associated with varying degrees of intralobular inflammatory infiltration. In some cases, bile duct lesions occur, which have been shown to be associated with a bad prognosis.

Furthermore, continuing necrosis and inflammation entail increasing fibrogenesis in the form of septal fibrosis which, together with parenchymal regeneration, causes progressive architectural disturbance eventually resulting in cirrhosis.

The simultaneous occurrence of a large variety of tissular changes creates great difficulty for adequate estimation of the degree of disease activity in CAH. Nevertheless, the formulation given in Table 1 gives an approximate idea of the location of a particular patient along the continuous spectrum of lesions in CAH. In the next section, a short description is given of the elementary lesions in CAH.

Piecemeal Necrosis (PMN). This term indicates liver-cell disappearance in close association with mononuclear inflammatory cell infiltration. The basic phenomenon thus is similar to that of "spotty necrosis". However, the term piecemeal necrosis has classically been applied to such lymphocyte-associated liver cell degeneration at the interface of interstitium and parenchyma.

The interface between normal interstitium and parenchyma refers to periportal piecemeal necrosis ("periportal hepatitis") (Popper and Schaffner 1971), associated with erosion of the limiting plate, whereas the interface between newly formed interstitium and parenchyma corresponds to periseptal (and hence intralobular) piecemeal necrosis (Bianchi et al. 1977).

The cellular infiltrate in piecemeal necrosis comprises a heterogeneous population of inflammatory cells, in which not only lymphocyte subsets can be identified, but also mononuclear cells which morphologically are identical to dentritic and interdigitating reticulum cells of lymphoid tissues; the latter are supposed to function as antigen-presenting cells (Desmet 1985). The predominant lymphocyte subset in piecemeal ne-

Table 1. Classification of chronic hepatitis

Category		Interstitium		Parenchyma		Architecture
CLH		Mild portal hepatitis·		Marked spotty necrosis		Normal
CPH		Portal hepatitis		Spotty necrosis		Normal
	Minimal		Minimal		Minimal	
	Marked		Marked		Marked	
Chronic septal hepatitis		Mild portal hepatitis		Minimal spotty necrosis		Passive septa—no nodules
NSRH		Mild (variable) portal hepatitis		Occasional spotty necrosis		Normal
				Kupffer cell activation		
CAH		PMN				
	Minimal		Mininal PMN	Mild spotty necrosis		Normal
	Moderate		Moderate PMN	Marked spotty necrosis		± Disturbed
	Severe		Severe PMN	Severe spotty necrosis		Disturbed
			active septa	Focal confluent necrosis		
				Zonal confluent necrosis		
	Very severe		Severe PMN	BHN		
			active septa		– PC CN	
					– Panlobular CN	Severely disturbed
			Bile duct lesion		– MLN	
Cirrhosis						
	Active	PMN		CN		Nodules + active septa
	Inactive	Portal hepatitis		Spotty necrosis		Nodules + passive septa

crosis corresponds to OKT_8+ suppressor/cytotoxic lymphocytes (Frazer et al. 1985), but also mononuclear phagocytes may be involved in mediating parenchymal liver cell damage (Bernuau et al. 1984).

Liver-cell necrosis in areas of PMN is thought to occur by apoptosis, i.e. fragmentation and disintegration of the hepatocyte (Kerr et al. 1979).

The contact between lymphocytes and parenchymal cells may be so close that lymphocytes are lying inside parenchymal liver cells: a feature termed emperipolesis (Bechtelsheimer et al. 1976).

In parenchymal areas "invaded" by PMN, liver cells at the invading frontier may become surrounded by lymphocytes, and sequestrated from the remaining part of the liver-cell plates (trapping of hepatocytes). Such sequestrated liver-cell groups often acquire a swollen, pale appearance, and group themselves around a central lumen: liver-cell rosettes. They become surrounded by collagen fibres (pericellular fibrosis) and are interpreted as attempts at regeneration in an unfavorable environment. Other liver cells show an increased eosinophilia and granularity, due to an increased number of mitochondria (mitochondriosis), comparable to oncocytes in other organs, and are indicated by the term oncocytic or acidophilic change (Lefkowitch et al. 1980).

Confluent Necrosis (CN) (Bianchi et al. 1971). Confluent necrosis refers to necrosis of groups of liver cells; the necrosis is of lytic type, with disappearance ("drop-out") of the affected parts of the parenchyma. This leads to denudation of the reticulin framework, which may collapse if the necrosis affects larger areas. Scavenger cells clear the cell debris (ceroid macrophages). According to its extent, CN may be graded as focal CN, zonal CN, portal-central CN, panlobular and multilobular necrosis (MLN).

Confluent necrosis seems to occur preferentially in the microcirculatory periphery of the liver units, leading to portal-central bridging necrosis when CN is located in the microcirculatory periphery (zone III) of simple acini (Bianchi et al. 1977). Panlobular necrosis refers to lytic necrosis of a whole liver lobule. Multilobular necrosis (Baggenstoss et al. 1972) affects several adjacent liver lobules, and apparently corresponds to CN in a whole acinar agglomerate (Rappaport 1976). The term bridging nepatic necrosis (BHN) has been proposed (Conn 1976; Boyer 1976) to indicate confluent necrosis linking portal tracts and central veins. BHN thus encompasses in increasing degree of severity portal-central confluent necrosis, panlobular, and multilobular necrosis.

Regeneration of Liver Cells. Regeneration of liver cells may be reflected in various appearances: actual liver-cell mitoses; appearance of small basophilic liver cells at the edge of CN; appearance of double cell thick plates; nodular regeneration; and in some instances appearance of multinucleated parenchymal giant cells.

Bile Duct Lesion (Poulsen and Christoffersen 1972). A peculiar lesion of interlobular bile ducts has been described in chronic hepatitis, usually in more severe variants. This lesion is seen in portal tracts with severe portal infiltration, often with lymphfollicle formation. The affected duct shows swelling and stratification of its lining cells, with permeation of lymphocytes and mononuclear cells in between. The basement membrane remains intact. In some cases it may be difficult to differentiate from bile duct lesions in primary biliary cirrhosis (PBC).

Fibrosis and Septum Formation. Fibrosis in chronic hepatitis is mostly of the septal type. Septal fibrosis may occur as active and passive septa (Bianchi et al. 1971).

Active septa correspond to connective tissue sheets, rich in inflammatory cell infiltration, and accompanied by PMN at their interface with the parenchyma. They are thought to originate from extensive PMN, invading in a wedge-shaped fashion into the parenchyma and eventually leading to portal-portal bridging (Bianchi et al. 1977), or by extension of PMN along areas of CN carrying the inflammatory cell populations deep into the lobules.

Passive septa correspond to connective tissue sheets carrying few or no inflammatory cells (paucicellular septa) and being sharply delineated at their interface from the parenchyma. They are mainly derived from post-necrotic collapse and scarring of areas of CN. Thus the topography of passive septa is largely determined by the topography of the preceding CN: e.g., portal-central septa derive from portal-central confluent necrosis (bridging hepatic necrosis). Active septa, in which the inflammatory activity fades out, acquire the appearance of paucicellular passive septa.

Multilobular CN leads to extensive areas of post-necrotic scarring, in which the approximated pre-existing portal tracts may still remain identifiable.

Cirrhosis. All forms of CAH may heal, but may also lead to cirrhosis in a substantial number of patients: slowly over the years with lower frequency in moderate CAH; more rapidly and in a higher number of cases in severe CAH.

The resulting cirrhosis is usually of the macronodular type. Cirrhosis represents the end evolutionary phase in the course of CAH, brought about by relentless inflammation and parenchymal destruction, counteracted by nodular regeneration.

Once the cirrhotic stage is reached, disease activity in terms of PMN and CN may continue, speeding up the fatal outcome (active cirrhosis), or may burn out, establishing a quiescent state in a structurally and hemodynamically altered liver (inactive cirrhosis). Inactive cirrhosis is characterized by paucicellular septa, sharp delineation between connective tissue and parenchyma (absence of PMN) and near-normal appearance of the nodular parenchyma. Active cirrhosis, on the contrary, features PMN at interstitial-parenchymal interfaces, and clearcut parenchymal lesions, including CN, in the nodules.

Thus in cirrhosis resulting from chronic hepatitis, disease activity is reflected by tissular changes similar to those in noncirrhotic chronic hepatitis.

Liver biopsy evaluation in chronic hepatitis should try to specify not only the degree of disease activity, but also the stage of structural derangement of lobular architecture. The latter may be difficult to recognize in needle specimens in macronodular cirrhosis, emphasizing the usefulness of laparoscopy (Semary et al. 1984).

4 Etiological Markers

Histological and immunohistochemical markers are helpful in establishing etiology in several cases of chronic hepatitis. In recent years, in situ hybridization techniques have further extended the possibility of etiological diagnosis.

Hepatitis B virus can be identified as the etiological agent in tissue sections by the finding of GGH (Hadziyannis 1981) and sanded nuclei (Bianchi and Gudat 1976). Immunohistochemical techniques (fluorescence, peroxidase) are more sensitive for detection of HBsAg and HBcAg. Processing of the liver specimen influences the sensitivity of immunohistochemical detection of HBcAg (Gowans and Burrel 1985). In situ hybridization to detect HBV-DNA sequences in chronically infected livers is helpful in elucidating the replicating strategy of the HBV genome and the mechanisms of hepatocyte injury (Burrel 1984; Burrel et al. 1984). Hepatitis B core antigen appears to be the target antigen for immune elimination of HBV-replicating hepatocytes (Alberti et al. 1984; Mandelli et al. 1984) (Vento et al. 1985).

Non-A, non-B hepatitis is reported to be characterized by mild fatty change, abundance of acidophil bodies, dense intralobular lymphocytic infiltration, parenchymal giant cells and the hepatitic type of bile duct lesion (Bianchi and Gudat 1983). Recent investigation, however, concluded that no single pathognomonic lesion exists that allows a reliable distinction to be made of hepatitis non-A, non-B from hepatitis A and B (Spichtin 1985; Vanstapel et al. 1986). Ultrastructural changes described in nuclei and cytoplasm of hepatocytes in non-A, non-B hepatitis still lack confirmation of specificity (Spichtin 1985; Desmet and De Vos 1985).

Delta hepatitis can be recognized on liver tissue sections by immunohistochemical demonstration of hepatitis delta antigen (Rizzetto and Verme 1985; Stöcklin et al. 1981). Delta infection in chronically HBV-infected patients is usually characterized by more severe intralobular and portal inflammatory changes (Lok et al. 1985).

Drug-induced chronic hepatitis may be suspected of the ground of eosinophil infiltration, cholestasis and granulomas (Bianchi et al. 1974).

Wilson's disease should be suspected when steatosis, glycogen nuclei, Mallory bodies, and copper accumulation are observed, especially in younger patients.

Alpha-1 antitrypsin (AAT) deficiency is recognized by characteristic PAS-positive hepatocellular inclusions in acinar zone 1 hepatocytes; these inclusions show specific AAT-immunoreactivity.

5 Histological Assessment of Activity

As described above, disease activity is expressed by the histological changes mentioned before, of which PMN and CN represent the most significant features.

It remains difficult, however, to assess degrees of disease activity from lengthy morphological descriptions. Attempts have been made to quantitate these lesions in numerical scores (Demeulenaere et al. 1981) and to express this evaluation by a Histological Activity Index (HAI) (Knodell et al. 1981).

HAI, when consistently reproducible by different observers, may prove useful in comparative studies of therapeutic results, expecially in cases with mild CAH, in which histological damage is not clearly reflected in clinical and biochemical symptoms.

Problems remain, however, since the scores of the HAI are arbitrary values attributed to histological changes, of which the intrinsic biological impact cannot be quantitatively measured; furthermore it is difficult to find an adequate numerical score which exactly weighs not only the amount of fibrosis, but also its topographical pattern. The topographical pattern of fibrosis (e.g., including portal-central septa which create the possibility for portal-central shunting and its functional and hemodynamic consequences) may be more important from a physio-pathological point of view than the total amount of fibrosis per se.

References

Alberti A, Trevisan A, Fattovich G, Realdi G (1984) The role of hepatitis B virus replication and hepatocyte membrane expression in the pathogenesis of HBV-related hepatic damage. In: Chisari FV (ed) Advances in hepatitis research. Masson, New York, pp 134–143

Baggenstoss AH, Soloway RD, Summerskill WHJ (1972) Chronic active liver disease: the range of histologic lesions, the response to treatment and evolution. Hum Pathol 3: 183–198

Bechtelsheimer H, Gedigk P, Müller R, Klein H (1976) Aggressive Emperipolese bei chronischen Hepatitiden. Klin Wochenschr 54: 137–140

Bernuau D, Rogier E, Feldman G (1984) In situ ultrastructural detection and quantitation of liver mononuclear phagocytes in contact with hepatocytes in chronic type B hepatitis. Lab Invest 51: 667–674

Bianchi L (1983) Liver biopsy interpretation in hepatitis. Part II. Histopathology and classification of acute and chronic viral hepatitis. Differential diagnosis. Pathol Res Pract 178: 180–213

Bianchi L, Gudat F (1976) Sanded nuclei in hepatitis B. Eosinophilic inclusions in liver cell nuclei due to excess in hepatitis B core antigen formation. Lab Invest 35: 1–5

Bianchi L, Gudat F (1983) Histo- and immunopathology of viral hepatitis. In: Deinhardt F, Deinhardt J (eds) Viral hepatitis: Laboratory and clinical sciences. Dekker, New York, pp 335–382

Bianchi L, De Groote J, Desmet VJ, Gedigk P, Korb G, Popper H, Poulsen H, Scheuer PJ, Schmid M, Thaler H, Wepler W (1971) Morphological criteria in viral hepatitis. Lancet i: 333–337

Bianchi L, De Groote J, Desmet VJ, Gedigk P, Korb G, Popper H, Poulsen H, Scheuer PJ, Schmid M, Thaler H, Wepler W (1974) Guidelines for diagnosis of therapeutic drug-induced liver injury in liver biopsies. Lancet i: 854–857

Bianchi L, De Groote J, Desmet VJ, Gedigk P, Korb G, Popper H, Poulsen H, Scheuer PJ, Schmid M, Thaler H, Wepler W (1977) Acute and chronic hepatitis revisited. Lancet ii: 914–919

Boyer JL (1976) Chronic hepatitis–a perspective on classification and determinants of prognosis. Gastroenterology 70: 1161–1171

Burrel CJ (1984) Cell-virus relationships in persistent hepatitis B infection in man: implications from in situ hybridisation studies. In: Chisari FV (ed) Advances in hepatitis research. Masson, New York, pp 62–68

Burrel CJ, Gowans EJ, Rowland R, Hall P, Jilbert AR, Marmion BP (1984) Correlation between liver histology and markers of hepatitis B virus replication: a study by in situ hybridisation. Hepatology 4: 20–24

Chadwick RG, Galizzi JJr, Heathcote J, Lyssiotis T, Cohen BJ, Scheuer PJ, Sherlock S (1979) Chronic persistent hepatitis: hepatitis B virus markers and histological follow up. Gut 20: 372–377

Conn HO (1976) Chronic hepatitis: reducing an iatrogenic enigma to a workable puzzle. Gastroenterology 70: 1182–1184

Degott C, Potet F (1983) Intérêts de la ponction-biopsie hépatique dans le diagnostic, le classement et le traîtement des hépatites chroniques. Ann Pathol 3: 5–18

De Groote J, Desmet VJ, Gedigk P, Korb G, Popper H, Poulsen H, Scheuer P, Schmid M, Thaler H, Uehlinger E, Wepler W (1968) A classification of chronic hepatitis. Lancet ii: 626–628

De Groote J, Fevery J, Lepoutre L (1978) Long-term follow-up of chronic active hepatitis of moderate severity. Gut 19: 510–513

Demeulenaere F, Desmet VJ, Dupont E, Fiasse R, Gisselbrecht H, Heully F, Jeanpierre R, Lecompte J, Lennes G, Macinot C, Migeotte P, Pirotte J, Rauber G, Ruyters L, Van Cauwenberge H (1981) Effects du (+)-cyanidanol-3 dans le traîtement de l'hépatite chronique active. Gastroenterol Clin Biol 5: 314–323

Desmet VJ (1985) New aspects of piecemeal necrosis. In: Bianchi L, Gerok W, Popper H (eds) Trends in hepatology. MTP Press, Lancaster, pp 183–200

Desmet VJ, De Vos R (1985) Ultrastructural findings in non-A, non-B viral hepatitis. In: Brunner H, Thaler H (eds) Hepatology: a Festschrift for Hans Popper. Raven, New York, pp 159–175

Frazer IH, Mackay IR, Bell J, Becker G (1985) The cellular infiltrate in the liver in auto-immune chronic active hepatitis: analysis with monoclonal antibodies. Liver 5: 162–172

Gerber MA, Vernace S (1974) Chronic septal hepatitis. Virchows Arch (A) 353: 303–309

Gowans EJ, Burrell CJ (1985) Widespread presence of cytoplasmic HBcAg in hepatitis B-infected liver detected by improved immunochemical methods. J Clin Pathol 38: 393–398

Hadziyannis SJ (1981) The ground-glass hepatocyte: an aid to diagnosis, a challenge to pathophysiology. In: Berk PD, Chalmers TC (eds) Frontiers in liver disease. Grune & Stratton, New York, pp 106–121

Kerr JFR, Searle J, Halliday WJ, Roberts I, Cooksley WGE, Halliday JW, Holder L, Burnett W, Powell LW (1979) The nature of piecemeal necrosis in chronic active hepatitis. Lancet ii: 827–828

Knodell RG, Ishak HG, Black WC, Chen TS, Craig R, Kaplowitz N, Kiernan TW, Wollman J (1981) Formulation and application of a numerical scoring system for assessing histological activity in asymptomatic chronic active hepatitis. Hepatology 1: 431–435

Lefkowitch JH, Arborgh BAM, Scheuer PJ (1980) Oxyphilic granular hepatocytes. Mitochondrion-rich liver cells in hepatic disease. Am J Clin Pathol 74: 432–441

Lenoir C, Buffet C, Martin E, Etienne JP (1978) Etude comparée des critères biologiques et histologiques au cours des hépatites chroniques. Proposition d'un classement des lésions histologiques en grades. Gastroenterol Clin Biol 2: 153–164

Liaw YF, Chu CM, Chen TJ, Lin DY, Chang-Chien CS, Wu CS (1982) Chronic lobular hepatitis: a clinicopathological and prognostic study. Hepatology 2: 258–262

Liaw YF, Sheen IS, Chu CM, Chen TJ (1984) Chronic hepatitis with nonspecific histological changes. Is it a distinct variant of chronic hepatitis? Liver 4: 55–60

Lok ASF, Lindsay I, Scheuer PJ, Thomas HC (1985) Clinical and histological features of delta infection in chronic hepatitis B virus carriers. J Clin Pathol 38: 530–533

Popper H, Schaffner F (1971) The vocabulary of chronic hepatitis. N Engl J Med 284: 1154–1156

Popper H, Schaffner F (1976) Chronic hepatitis: Taxonomic, etiologic and therapeutic problems. In: Popper H, Schaffner F (eds) Progress in liver disease, vol V. Grune & Stratton, New York, pp 531–558

Poulsen H, Christoffersen P (1972) Abnormal bile duct epithelium in chronic aggressive hepatitis and cirrhosis. A review of morphology and clinical, biochemical and immunologic features. Human Pathol 3: 217–225

Rappaport AM (1976) The microcirculatory acinar concept of normal and pathological hepatic structure. Beitr Pathol 157: 215–243

Rizzetto M, Verme G (1985) Review. Delta hepatitis–present status. J Hepatol 1: 187–193

Scheuer PJ (1977) Chronic hepatitis: a problem for the pathologist. Histopathology 1: 5–19

Semary M, Geubel AP, Rahier J, Belassai J, Jamart J, Dive C (1984) Chronic active hepatitis (CAH). The diagnostic and prognostic value of laparoscopy. Acta Gastro-Enterol Belg 47: 490–499

Spichtin HP (1985) Hepatitis non-A, non-B (NANB): epidemiologische, klinische, serologische und morphologische Aspekte. Klin Wochenschr 63: 289–404

Stöcklin E, Gudat F, Krey G, Dürmüller U, Gasser M, Schmid M, Stalder G, Bianchi L (1981) Delta antigen in hepatitis B: immunohistology of frozen and paraffin-embedded liver biopsies and relation to HBV-infection. Hepatology 1: 238–242

Thaler H (1974) The natural history of chronic hepatitis. In: Schaffner F, Sherlock S. Leevy CM (eds) The liver and its diseases. Thieme, Stuttgart, pp 207–215

Vanstapel MJ, Rugge M, Fevery J, De Roo D, De Groote J, Guido M, Realdi G, Tremolada F, Desmet V (1986) In search for histological characteristics for chronic non-A, non-B hepatitis, in comparison with chronic hepatitis B infection. In: Liaw Y-F (ed) Proceedings of the International Symposium on Chronic Hepatitis, Taipei, 18-29 Nov. 1985. Elsevier Science Publishers (in press)

Vento S, Hegarty JE, Alberti A, O'Brien CJ, Alexander GJM, Eddleston ALWF, Williams R (1985) T lymphocyte sensitization to HBcAg and T cell-mediated unresponsiveness to HBsAg in Hepatitis B virus-related chronic liver disease. Hepatology 5: 192–197

Prognostic Significance of Viral Antigens in Liver Tissue

F. CALLEA, F. FACCHETTI, E. BONERA, G. GRASSO CAPRIOLI, and M. ZORZI[1]

1 Introduction

Over the past 15 years, a number of observations have culminated in the localization of viral antigens in liver tissue by the use of routine histology, immunohistochemistry, electron microscopy (EM), and immuno-electron microscopy (IEM).

Routine histology has proved to be useful in conditions of massive intracellular content of hepatitis B surface antigen (HBsAg), resulting in a ground-glass (G-G) appearance of the hepatocytic cytoplasm (Hadziyannis et al. 1973); in rare instances, excess formation of core antigen (HBcAg) particles in the nuclei has been correlated with a "sanded" appearance in hematoxylin eosin-(H.E.)-stained preparations (Bianchi and Gudat 1976).

In contrast to HBsAg and HBcAg, delta as well as NA-NB viruses do not result in any peculiar cytological change.

On H.E.-stained sections, HBsAg-G-G hepatocytes cannot be differentiated from similar cells occurring in conditions other than HBV infection. This topic has been recently reviewed (Callea et al. 1986).

Although a number of empiric stains, among others orcein (Shikata et al. 1974) and Victoria blue (Tanaka et al. 1981), are available for differentiating HBsAg-G-G hepatocytes, specific characterization requires the use of immunohistochemistry, EM, or IEM.

EM has revealed the morphology of both HBsAg and HBcAg particles, but it has been found useless for identification of NA-NB or delta agents. Ultrastructural changes in the latter conditions lack specificity (De Vos et al. 1983; Kamimura et al. 1983). IEM has played an important role not only in specific characterization of particulate-HBV antigens (Yamada and Nakane 1977; Yamada et al. 1978), but also in indirect visualization of nonparticulate-viral antigens, including HBcAg (Kojima 1982) and delta-Ag (Kojima et al. 1985).

EM and IEM, together with identification of specific HB-associated antigen and antibodies in blood, supplemented by in vitro measurements of cellular immunity, have greatly enhanced our knowledge of the natural history of HB.

In this paper we discuss the role of immunohistochemistry in the diagnosis of viral hepatitis B, with special reference to the prognostic significance of HBsAg, HBcAg and

---

1 Histochemistry Unit 1st Department of Pathology, and 3rd Department of Internal Medicine, Spedali Civili of Brescia, 25100 Brescia, Italy

Viral Hepatitis, ed. by F. Callea et al.
© Springer-Verlag Berlin Heidelberg 1986

delta-Ag patterns in liver tissue. For this purpose, we have reviewed a series of liver biopsy specimens from 250 HBsAg-positive cases collected in the Department of Pathology of Brescia Hospital.

2 Immunohistochemical Detection of Viral Antigens in Liver Tissue

Original work on tissue localization of HBV and delta antigens was carried out by the immunofluorescence technique (Coyne et al. 1970; Gudat et al. 1975; Rizzetto et al. 1977). Since then immunoperoxidase techniques have become largely available. The latter are more sensitive and permanent-staining techniques; moreover immunoperoxidase-stained sections can be counterstained with hematoxylin for the simultaneous evaluation of both viral antigens distribution and histological features. Furthermore, double or triple immunoperoxidase stains have been successively applied on a single tissue section for the simultaneous visualization of two or three antigens (Huang and Neurath 1979; Facchetti et al. 1986).

Our immunohistochemical study was carried out with a conventional peroxidase-antiperoxidase (PAP) technique (Facchetti et al. 1986) applied on paraffin-embedded or frozen-liver biopsy specimens; in addition, the more sensitive avidin-biotin peroxidase complex technique according to Hsu et al. (1981) was used for selected cases.

Serial sections alternately or successively stained for HBsAg, HBcAg, and delta-Ag were scrutinized to determine: (A) cellular localization, (B) simultaneous presence, and (C) expression patterns, indicative of etiology, prognosis, and pathogenesis.

2.1 Cellular Localization of Viral Antigens

HBsAg was demonstrated in the cytoplasm and/or on the plasma membrane of hepatocytes. Cytoplasmic positive staining could be focal, submembraneous, or diffuse. The diffuse type was often associated with a G-G appearance, but in cases with a low intracellular antigen charge, it could also be found in cells lacking peculiar cytological changes. Demonstration of membrane-associated HBsAg was easier in frozen than in paraffin-embedded tissue.

HBcAg was demonstrated in the nuclei, cytoplasm, and on the plasma membrane of liver cells. In 10 out of 250 cases, cytoplasmic core was detected in hepatocytes with a G-G appearance in the absence of HBsAg. This new variant of G-G hepatocyte (HBcAg-G-G) was first reported in delta-positive cases from this study material (Facchetti et al. 1986).

The demonstration of cytoplasmic and/or membrane-associated HBcAg was easier in frozen than in paraffin-embedded tissue. The more sensitive avidin-biotin peroxidase technique made it possible to detect very small amounts of both HBsAg and HBcAg in the hepatocytic cytoplasm from a few paraffin sections which had been negative with the conventional PAP technique (see sect. 2.3.3 and 2.3.4). Delta-Ag was found mostly in the nuclei and rarely in the cytoplasm (Kojima et al. 1985; Facchetti et al. 1986). E-Ag was not sought in this study. Previous works have claimed a cytoplasmic localization for e-Ag (Trepo et al. 1976), whilst others reported a nuclear posi-

Table 1. Cellular localization of viral antigens

Antigen	Nuclei	Cytopl.	Membrane
HBsAg	–	+	+
HBcAg	+	+	+
Delta-Ag	+	+	?
e-Ag	+	+	?

tivity (Arnold et al. 1977); more recently, e-Ag has been demonstrated by IEM in both nuclei and cytoplasm (Kojima 1982). The cellular localization of viral antigens is summarized in Table 1.

2.2 Simultaneous Presence of Viral Antigens

HBsAg and HBcAg occurred simultaneously in 126 out of 250 cases; HBsAg and delta-Ag were found simultaneously in 42 cases, 7 of which displayed also HBcAg. In 65 cases, HBsAg was detected in the absence of either core or delta. In 3 cases only delta was demonstrated; the remaining 14 cases were negative.

Two or three antigens could be demonstrated in the same cell under the following combination: nuclear and membrane HBcAg + cytoplasmic HBsAg; nuclear delta + cytoplasmic core; nuclear delta and core; cytoplasmic delta and HBsAg; (very rarely) binucleated hepatocytes with delta or core in each nucleus + HBsAg in the cytoplasm.

Cumulative results are summarized in Tables 2 and 3. Quantitative estimation of HBcAg was referred to as focal or generalized, according to Bianchi and Gudat (1976).

Table 2. Immunohistochemical results for HBsAg, HBcAg, and delta-Ag in 250 cases

HBsAg + HBcAg + delta-Ag	7
HBsAg + delta-Ag	35
HBsAg + HBcAg	126
HBsAg	65
Delta-Ag	3
Negative	14

Table 3. Simultaneous occurrence of viral antigens in a single cell

Nucleus/Cytopl.	Cytopl./Cytopl.	Nucleus/Nucleus
HBcAg/HBsAg	HBcAg/HBsAg	Delta/HBcAg
Delta/HBsAg	Delta/HBsAg	
Delta/HBcAg		
HBcAg/HBsAg		
+		
Delta		

2.3 Expression Patterns of Viral Antigens

In 1975 Gudat et al. forwarded a biological classification of HB based upon the recognition of four patterns of HBsAg and HBcAg in the liver: (1) focal HBcAg type, (2) generalized HBcAg type, (3) HBcAg-free HBsAg type, (4) elimination type (absence of both HBsAg and HBcAg). Each of these proved to have a different diagnostic and prognostic implication. This classification was correlated with conventional histological diagnosis, thus indicating an intrinsic association between the type and degree of inflammation and the stage of viral replication (Bianchi and Gudat 1979).

Bianchi's classification is still valid as far as it went. Since then delta has been discovered; moreover, additional immunohistochemical expression patterns for HBsAg and HBcAg (Negro et al. 1984; Bonino et al. 1986; Tardanico et al. 1985) have been identified. It seemed timely, therefore, to review the whole subject.

In our series the following expression patterns of HBsAg, HBcAg, and delta-Ag were observed: (1) presence of HBsAg and HBcAg, (2) cytoplasmic HBcAg, (3) absence of HBsAg and HBcAg, (4) presence of HBsAg in the absence of HBcAg, (5) presence of delta-Ag.

Correlation of immunohistochemical results and liver morphology led us to propose a simplified classification of antigen expressions into: nonaggressive and aggressive patterns.

1. Presence of HBsAg and HBcAg. In Bianchi's classification, liver biopsy specimens containing both HBsAg and HBcAg were separated into two different groups: the generalized core type, having HBcAg in the vast majority of liver cell nuclei (up to 100%); and the focal core type, having spotty representation of nuclear HBcAp (up to 60%). Presence of HBcAg was referred to as purely nuclear and no specific mention of cytoplasmic localization was made. In both types, cytoplasmic HBsAg was observed in about 20–30% of hepatocytes. Membrane-associated HBsAg was frequently seen in the focal type but was impressive (so-called honeycomb pattern) in the generalized type.

These two patterns were associated with different liver histology: the focal type occurred in chronic aggressive hepatitis (CAH), acute hepatitis with signs of transition to chronicity (AHTC), and active cirrhosis. The generalized type was found in livers with no inflammation at all, or with mild nonaggressive inflammation (HBcAg carriers). Generalized core was a characteristic finding in efficiently immunosuppressed patients (e.g., kidney transplant recipients) (Gudat et al. 1975), in children born to HBsAg-positive mothers (vertical transmission) (Dunn et al. 1972; Schweitzer et al. 1973), in cancer patients (Nowoslawski et al. 1970), in patients on long-term treatment with cytostatic and/or immunesuppressive agents, and in individuals without overt immune deficiency (spontaneous carriers) (Bianchi and Gudat 1979).

In our study, the presence of HBcAg was invariably associated with liver damage. Although in a few cases distinction between focal and generalized pattern was purely subjective, as a general rule, liver damage was, according to Bianchi, mild in cases with generalized core and more severe in cases with focal core.

The focal type of nuclear core was consistently associated with CAH. In addition, it occurred in three cases at the height of acute lobular hepatitis (ALH), in a few cases with features of later stages of AH or with milder forms of chronic hepatits, i.e., nonspecific reactive hepatitis (NSRH), chronic persistent hepatitis (CPH), chronic lobular (CLH) and chronic septal hepatitis (CSH). Interestingly, most of these cases showed clearcut evidence of piecemeal necrosis (CAH) when serial follow-up biopsy specimens were examined.

These observations support the interpretation of the focal type of nuclear core as a sign of aggressivity (aggressive pattern).

When the generalized type of nuclear core occurred in association with cytoplasmic expression of HBcAg, the corresponding liver histology was that of CAH (see Sect. 2.3.1), even in patients under immunosuppressive treatment.

2. Cytoplasmic Core. This pattern was not included in Bianchi's classification. Cytoplasmic HBcAg is now being observed with an increasing incidence (Yamada et al. 1978; Huang and Neurath 1979, Negro et al. 1984; Bonino et al. 1985; Gowans and Burrel 1985; Tardanico et al. 1985; Facchetti et al. 1986). In our study material cytoplasmic HBcAg appeared as either focal or generalized, eventually being associated with nuclear and/or membrane expression of core. Exclusive cytoplasmic HBcAg could also result in a G-G appearance of hepatocytes. All cases with cytoplasmic localization of HBcAg were associated with histological features of CAH and the staining pattern remained unchanged over the years, as documented in a series of follow-up biopsies. Nine of such cases presented HBV-DNA and anti-HB-e antibodies in serum. Similar features had previously been reported by Negro et al. (1984) and Bonino et al. (1985). CAH with cytoplasmic core in the liver and HBV-DNA and anti-e antibodies in the serum appears to represent a separate entity of chronic hepatitis with an unfavorable prognosis (Bonino et al. 1985). Clinical pathological features of this disease entity are summarized in Table 4.

Recently, other authors (Kojima and Desmet 1984), in an IEM study, have reported cytoplasmic core as the main staining pattern in liver biopsies with severe liver cell damage, while in cases with minimal parenchymal damage the presence of HBcAg was restricted to the nuclei. These observations point to cytoplasmic core pattern as a sign of chronic active liver diseases (aggressive pattern). Further practical details of diagnostic utility on focal nuclear core and on cytoplasmic core patterns are mentioned below (see Sect. 2.3.4).

Table 4. HBV-DNA, anti-HBe Chronic
hepatitis: clinical pathological features

---

1. CAH
2. Unfavorable prognosis
3. Cytoplasmic core pattern
4. Staining pattern persists in serial
   follow-up biopsies

---

3. Absence of HBsAg and HBcAg. In Bianchi's classification this condition was referred to as elimination type because it occurred in AL self-limited hepatitis. In our series, 20 cases were negative for both HBcAg and HBsAg in liver sections stained with the conventional PAP technique. On routine histology, 9 of these cases showed features of steatosis and/or mild fibrosis of alcoholic type in the absence of significant inflammation; the remaining 11 cases showed features of ALH. In 3 out of 9 alcoholic cases, a cytoplasmic positive staining for HBsAg, but not for HBcAg, was found in a few hepatocytes (spotty representation), when sections were stained with the more sensitive avidin-biotin technique. These 3 patients were consequently classified as healthy HBsAg carriers (see Sect. 2.3.4).

The discrepancy between serum positivity and tissue negativity for HBsAg can be explained either by the higher sensitivity of RIA as compared to immunohistochemistry, or by sampling error, particularly in cases with spotty representation of low amounts of antigen.

Among 11 ALH cases showing the elimination type pattern when sought for HBsAg and HBcAg, 3 cases did not recover. On serial follow-up biopsy specimens obtained a few months and a few years later, these three cases presented features of CLH and finally of delta-positive CAH. Previous biopsy specimens were therefore retrospectively examined for delta-Ag, which was indeed found in all cases including the original specimens. These cases, consequently classified as delta hepatitis, emphasize the potentiality of delta-Ag in determining the transition of acute into chronic hepatitis.

In contrast to the elimination type pattern, the finding of HBcAg and/or HBsAg expressions in a liver biopsy at the height of ALH indicates viral elimination insufficiency. Likewise the finding of viral expressions in later stages of AH indicates persistence, even if histological signs of chronicity are not present in the biopsy (see Sect. 2.3.1, and Bianchi and Gudat 1979).

4. Presence of HBsAg in the Absence of HBcAg. The presence of HBsAg in the absence of core (HBcAg-free HBsAg type) in Bianchi's classification was characteristic of the healthy carrier state and of nonaggressive liver diseases. This pattern was found in normal or early normal livers and in cases with nonaggressive forms of hepatitis: NSRH, CPH, or inactive cirrhosis.

In our study 108 cases were found to be positive for HBsAg but negative for core. Only 40 cases, however, fitted into the HBcAg-free HBsAg type: 30 showed a nearly normal liver (HBsAg carriers) and 10 presented inactive cirrhosis (7 of them had concomitant HCC). The remaining 68 cases were CAH. This observation stimulated an extensive investigation to clarify the relationship between HBV infection and CAH in these 68 cases.

Sensitivity of the technique and sampling error were found to be responsible for HBcAg-negative staining in 8 cases. Indeed, 4 cases which had been negative in paraffin sections with the conventional PAP method revealed a cytoplasmic positive staining for core with the more sensitive avidin-biotin technique; furthermore, 4 cases which had been negative in paraffin sections revealed a positive staining for core in a few nuclei when additional frozen-stored material from the same cases was examined. Thus these 8 cases proved to be authentic type-B CAH with immunohistochemical aggressive patterns.

Thirty five of the remaining 60 cases were positive on staining for delta, and consequently classified as delta-CAH (see Sect. 2.3.5).

Among the remaining 25 cases with HBsAg positivity in the absence of demonstrable HBcAg or delta-Ag, two distinct subgroups have emerged in which chronic liver disease was apparently not related to HBV but was rather due to associated pathology. Seven were alcoholics (chronic alcoholic hepatitis in HBsAg carriers), two cases alpha-1-antitrypsin (AAT) deficiency (Pi MZ phenotype in HBsAg carriers).

A high incidence of AAT deficiency has been reported in cryptogenic cirrhosis and NB-CAH (Hodges et al. 1981). Our finding, i.e., AAT deficiency in HBsAg-positive patients, represents a new observation.

By staining immunohistochemically liver biopsy specimens in search of the Z allele of AAT (Callea et al. 1986), we were able to collect 7 such cases including 5 cases previously studied in association with Dr. V. Desmet (Callea 1983). That has provided the opportunity of detecting for the first time HBsAg and AAT in the same liver cells at both light and EM level (Fig. 1).

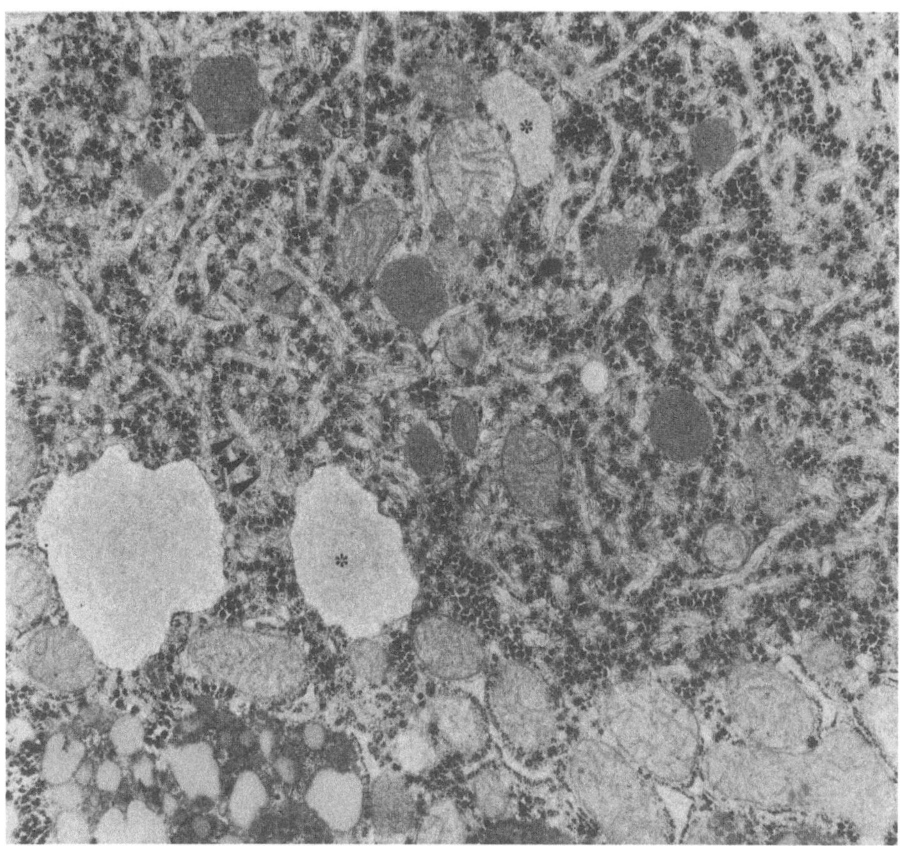

Fig. 1. Liver biopsy specimen from a HBsAg-positive Pi MZ phenotype patient. The electronmicrograph shows a portion of a hepatocyte with longitudinally cut tubules and cross-sectioned dots of HBsAg (⇒) in the cisternae of the SER. A few dilated cisternae of the RER contain AAT (*). x 23000

Table 5. HBcAg-free HBsAg pattern in CAH: spectrum of conditions

1. HBV:	– Sampling error (focal core) – Sensitivity of technique (cytoplasmic core)
2. Superinfection:	– Delta – Delta-like? – NA-NB?
3. Nonviral associated pathology:	– Alcohol – AAT Deficiency (Pi MZ phenotype)
4. Autoimmunity:	– Liver-cell neoantigens
5. Others	

In the remaining 16 cases, the etiology of CAH remained undetermined. One might speculate about a possible implication of superinfection by delta-like or NA-NB agents; unfortunately, specific markers for these etiologies are not available at present. Further, autoimmune mechanisms against plasma membrane neo-antigens might be considered, according to Arnold et al. (1977) and Meyer zum Buschenfelde et al. (1979).

The spectrum of conditions under which the so-called HBcAg-free HBsAg pattern occurs in histologically proved CAH is summarized in Table 5.

5. Presence of Delta-Ag. This condition was not included in Bianchi's classification. Delta infection worsens the course of viral hepatitis B (Smedile et al. 1982; Rizzetto et al. 1983). Recently, delta-Ag has also been implicated in epidemic fulminant hepatitis (Popper et al. 1983).

In acute infection delta is known to inhibit HBV replication (Rizzetto 1983), thus explaining the possibility of ALH resulting in the elimination type pattern.

In our series of 45 delta-positive cases, the role of delta in determining transition of AH into chronicity has been documented in 3 cases (see Sect. 2.3.3).

In chronic delta carriers, liver histology is usually that of CAH, with or without cirrhosis, and features of CLH are often present (Lock et al. 1985).

A mutual exclusion between HBcAg and delta is reported (Rizzetto et al. 1977; Canese et al. 1979; Verme et al. 1983). In our series 7 out of 45 cases (16%) presented both core and delta, in addition to HBsAg. Liver biopsy specimens from cases presenting both core and delta were characterized by features of a more severe CAH (3 cases also had cirrhosis) than those without HBcAg: very dense lymphoid aggregates in portal tracts and septa, pronounced periportal piecemeal necrosis, and marked intralobular activity (Table 6).

Presence of delta-Ag in the liver represents a further pattern of aggressivity.

Expressions of HBsAg and HBcAg in delta-positive biopsies have been reported in detail (Facchetti et al. 1986).

In summary, liver biopsy specimens from patients who are positive for HBsAg in serum, reveal various expression patterns when stained by immunohistochemical techniques for HBsAg, HBcAg, and delta-Ag.

A negative staining for these three antigens seems to be associated with two conditions: (1) acute lobular (AL) self-limited hepatitis or (2) low amounts of intrahepatic antigens.

The discrepancy between serum positivity and tissue negativity for HBsAg can be explained either by sampling error or by the higher sensitivity of the RIA method as compared with immunohistochemistry.

Table 6. Histological features in delta-positive CH

Histology	No. Cases	Delta + HBsAg	Delta + HBsAg + HBcAg
	42	35	7
Lymphoid aggregate		+	+ +
Piecemeal necrosis		+	+ +
Lobular activity		+ +	+ + +

In cases with a positive staining for viral antigens, two main patterns can be distinguished: nonaggressive and aggressive patterns.

The nonaggressive pattern is reflected in (a) the HBcAg-free HBsAg type (HBsAg carriers) or (b) the generalized type of nuclear core (HBcAg carriers).

The aggressive pattern is reflected in (c) presence of delta or (d) delta + core or (e) the focal type of nuclear core, or (f) the cytoplasmic core pattern.

Superinfection of HBsAg carriers, or switching from generalized to focal core, with or without cytoplasmic expression of HBcAg, results in transition from nonaggressive to aggressive pattern (Table 7).

The aggressive pattern occurs in association with histological features of CAH. When occurring in ALH cases or in milder forms of chronic hepatitis, evolution into CAH has to be expected (Table 8).

Features of severe CAH, eventually with cirrhosis, are found in association with two new expression patterns: the cytoplasmic core and the simultaneous presence of HBcAg and delta. When features of CAH are observed in liver specimens with HBcAg-free HBsAg type, the liver disease may be due to superinfection or to nonviral etiology (AAT deficiency is also a possibility).

Table 7. Possible mechanism of transition from nonaggressive to aggressive pattern

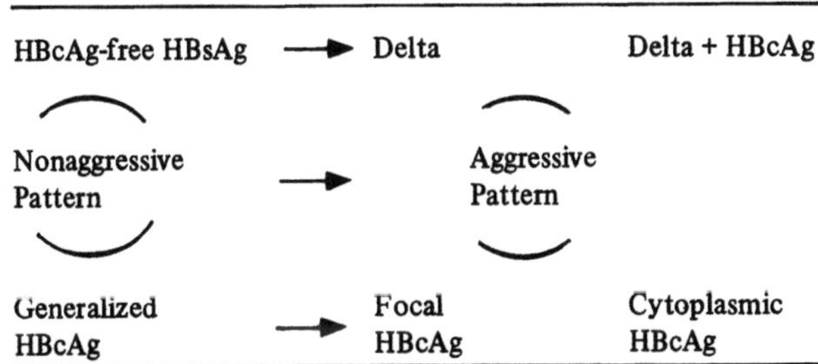

Table 8. Expression patterns under which transition from milder forms of chronic hepatitis into CAH occurs

Expression Patterns	Liver histology	Prognosis
Delta	ALH	
Delta + core	CLH	
Focal core	CPH	→ CAH
Cytoplasmic core	NSRH	
	CSH	

3 Pathogenesis of Liver-Cell Damage in Viral Hepatitis

The pathogenesis of liver-cell damage in viral hepatits is not entirely clarified. In contrast to delta (Rizzetto 1983; Popper et al. 1983), HBV seems to be of no, or only of a low grade, cytopathogenicity. This is best exemplified by HBsAg and HBcAg carriers, who tolerate large amounts of viral antigens in liver and blood without substantial liver-cell damage. Hepatocytic injury is believed to take place via immunological interactions with viral antigens on liver cells (Bianchi and Gudat 1979). Both HBcAg and HBsAg on liver cell membrane have been considered the target of immunological attack (Edgington and Chisari 1975; Gudat and Bianchi 1977b; Bianchi and Gudat 1979; Alberti et al. 1984; Mondelli et al. 1984).

We have been intrigued by the observation that HBsAg is expressed on the cell membrane not only in CAH (Nowoslawski et al. 1975; Ray et al. 1976; Huang and Neurath 1979), but mostly in patients who do not show signs of chronic inflammation, i.e., immunosuppressed kidney transplant recipients (Gudat et al. 1975), children born to HBsAg-positive mothers (Schweitzer et al. 1973), or even in healthy carriers (Furuta et al. 1975).

To try to clarify the significance of membrane-associated-HBsAg in the spectrum of HBV infection, Facchetti et al. (1985) investigated three groups of patients selected on the basis of a striking presence of HBsAg on the plasma membrane: one group was severe CAH, the two others had minor or no liver disease (i.e., kidney transplants and children born to HBsAg-positive mothers).

These three groups showed marked differences with regard to the immunohistochemical patterns of HBcAg and of major histocompatibility antigens (HLA) in liver cells (Table 9). HBcAg appeared as focal (aggressive pattern) in CAH, but it was absent or of generalized type (nonaggressive pattern) in the remaining two groups. HLA class I and II were expressed in very large amounts in hepatocytes from CAH cases, class I resulting in a striking "honeycomb" pattern. In transplants and children with vertical transmission, HLA class I was weakly expressed on the sinusoidal border ("sinusoidal" pattern). These results, schematically represented in Fig. 2, are interpreted to indicate that immunological elimination of cells displaying viral "target" antigens (including

Table 9. Relationship between expression of HBcAg, HBsAg, and HLA in CAH, transplants, and vertical transmission

	Memb. HBsAg	Hepatocytes			
		HBcAg		HLA	
		Foc/Abs/Gen		I	II
5 *CAH*	100%	*5*		*H*	++
6 Transpl.	100%	3	3	S	–
4 Vert. Transm.	100%	2	2	S	–

H = honeycomb; S = sinusoidal

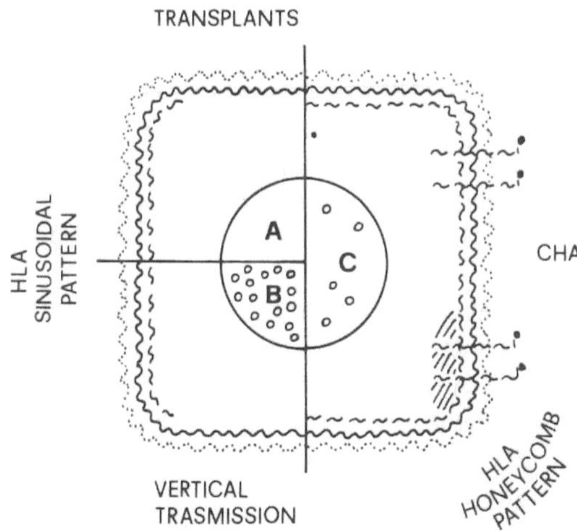

Fig. 2. Schematic representation of HBsAg, HBcAg, and HLA expressions in hepatocytes from transplants, vertical transmission and CAH. *A* and *B* nuclear patterns of HBcAg in transplants and in vertical transmission. *C* pattern of core in CAH. HBsAg (.....) is expressed on the cell membrane in *A*, *B*, and *C*. Very small amounts of HLA (- - - -) are expressed on the cell membrane in *A* and *B*, in the form of "sinusoidal" pattern. Enhanced expressions of HLA in the cytoplasm and cell membrane in the form of "honeycomb" pattern are found in *C* (CAH). HLA presents HBsAg (●●●) to the external surface for immunological interactions

HBsAg) on the cell membrane requires adequate expression of HLA on the plasma membrane in association with the focal type of nuclear core.

4 Expression of HBV Antigens in the Liver of HBsAg-Negative Patients

This possibility has recently been advanced by Brechot et al. (1985), who reported HBsAg-associated determinants in the liver and HBV-DNA sequences in the serum of patients with chronic liver disease and no HBV serological markers. The results from that study indicate a high frequence of HBsAg-negative HBV-DNA-positive viral infection of the liver and suggest that multiplication of HBV may occur in the absence of any conventional serological marker for HBV. Further investigations are needed to clarify this interesting observation.

5 Conclusions

Immunohistochemistry allows quantitative evaluation, simultaneous detection, and cellular localization of viral antigens in liver tissue. The various expression patterns appear to reflect the replication of viral agents and/or the state of specific immuneresponse. By correlating viral expressions with conventional histological diagnosis two main immunohistochemical patterns can be distinguished: nonaggressive and aggressive pattern.

The nonaggressive pattern results from the generalized type of nuclear core (HBcAg carrier) or from the so-called HBcAg-free HBsAg type (HBsAg carrier).

The aggressive pattern results from presence of delta, delta + core, focal type of nuclear core and cytoplasmic HBcAg pattern. Superinfection of HBsAg carrier or switching from generalized to focal core, with or without cytoplasmic expression of HBcAg, result in transition from nonaggressive to aggressive pattern.

Among the various described combinations, cytoplasmic core is most interesting for two main reasons; (1) biological and clinical implications, (2) morphological features.

Cytoplasmic core may partly reflect a primary synthesis of HBcAg in the cytoplasm. Nonparticulate-HBcAg is likely to be produced in the cytoplasm on ribosomes; subsequently it migrates into the nucleus for assembly into virus-like core particle (Yamada et al. 1978). Thereafter, presumably, core particles move through nuclear pores into the cytoplasm (De Vos et al. 1978), entering the cisternae of ER (where they are enveloped by HBsAg filaments to form complete virus or Dane particle) or are redistributed over the jaloplasm (Yamada et al. 1977; De Vos et al. 1978; Huang and Neurath 1979).

Different hypotheses have been advanced about the flow mechanism of core particles toward the plasma membrane (Gudat and Bianchi 1977a; Kojima and Desmet 1984).

On the clinical ground, cytoplasmic core is associated with a separate entity of chronic hepatitis, characterized by severe prognosis and presence in serum of both HBV-DNA and anti-e antibodies. The latter observation points to a correlation between immunohistochemistry and new diagnostic techniques provided by recombinant DNA.

On morphological ground, cytoplasmic core may result in a G-G appearance of the hepatocytic cytoplasm (HBcAg-G-G) which need not exhibit HBsAg. The precise subcellular localization, as well as the ultrastructural appearance of HBcAg in the newly described HBcAg-GG-hepatocytes are still to be determined.

The pathogenesis of liver cell damage is not fully established. Immunological mechanisms addressed against target-viral antigens on the cell membrane are most likely. However, elimination of infected cells requires not only the exposure of viral antigens but also additional microenvironmental factors, including enhanced expression of HLA on the cell membrane in combination with the focal type of nuclear core.

The final prognosis of HBV infection depends upon several interrelated events: superinfection, immunology, genetics including integration of HBV-DNA into the host genome, treatment, vaccination, and environmental factors, which are discussed elsewhere in this volume.

References

Alberti A, Trevisan A, Fattovich G, Realdi G (1984) The role of hepatitis B virus replication and hepatocyte membrane expression in the pathogenesis of HBV-related hepatic damage. In: Chisari FV (ed) Advances in hepatitis research. Masson, New York, pp 134–143

Arnold W, Nielsen JO, Hardts F, Meyer zum Buschenfelde KH (1977) Localization of e-antigen in nuclei of hepatocytes in HBsAg-positive liver disease. Gut 19: 994–996

Bianchi L, Gudat F (1976) Sanded nuclei in hepatitis B. Eosinophilic inclusions in liver cell nuclei due to excess in hepatitis B core antigen formation. Lab Invest 35: 1–5

Bianchi L, Gudat F (1979) Immunopathology of hepatitis B. In: Popper H, Schaffner F (eds) Progress in liver disease, vol VI. Grune & Stratton, New York, pp 371–392

Bonino F, Negro F, Tardanico R, Callea F, Verme G, Rizzetto M (1985) Chronic anti-HBe hepatitis with serum HBV-DNA. A separate entitiy. Hepatology 4: 1041

Bonino F, Rosina F, Rizzetto M, Rizzi R, Chiaberge E, Tardanico R, Callea F, Verme G (1986) Chronic hepatitis in HBsAg carriers with serum HBV-DNA and anti-HBe. Gastroenterology (in press)

Brechot, Degos F, Lugassy C, Thiers V, Zafrani S, Franco D, Bismuth H, Trepo C, Benhamou JP, Wands J, Isselbacher K, Tiollais P, Berthelot P (1985) Hepatitis B virus DNA in patients with chronic liver disease and negative tests for hepatitis B surface antigen. N Engl J Med 312: 270–276

Callea F (1983) Immunohistochemical study on alpha-1-antitrypsin. Thesis Acco, Leuven, pp 78–86

Callea F, De Vos R, Togni R, Tardanico R, Vanstapel MJ, Desmet VJ (1986) Fibrinogen inclusions in liver cells: a new type of ground-glass hepatocyte. Immune light and electron microscopic characterization. Histopathology 10: 65–73

Callea F, Fevery J, De Groote J, Desmet VJ (1986) Detection of Pi Z phenotype individuals by alpha-1-antitrypsin (AAT) immunohistochemistry in paraffin embedded liver specimens. J Hepatology 2: 389–401

Coyne (Zavatone) VE, Millman I, Cerda J, Gerstley BJS, London T, Sutnick A, Blumberb BS (1970) The localization of Australia Antigen by immunofluorescence. J Exp Med 131: 307–325

Canese MG, Rizzetto M, Aricò S, Crivelli O, Zanetti AR, Macchiorlati E, Ponzetto A, Leone L, Mollo F, Verme G (1979) An ultrastructural and immunohistochemical study on the antigen associated with the hepatitis B virus. J Pathol 128: 169–175

De Vos R, Ray MB, Desmet VJ (1978) Electron microscopy of hepatitis B virus components in chronic active liver disease. J Clin Pathol 32: 590–600

De Vos R, Vanstapel MJ, Desmyter J, De Wolf-Peeters, De Groote G, Colaert J. Mortelmnans J, De Groote J, Fevery J, Desmet V (1983) Are nuclear particles specific for non-A, non-B hepatitis? Hepatology 3: 532–544

Dunn AEG, Peters RL, Schwaitzer IL, Spears RL (1972) Virus-like particles in livers of infants with vertically transmitted hepatitis. Arch Pathol 94: 258

Edgington GS, Chisari FV (1975) Immunological aspects of hepatitis B virus infection. Am J Med Sci 270: 213–227

Facchetti F, Bonera E, Albertini A, Zorzi M, Callea F (1985) Immunohistochemical patterns of HBcAg, HLA class I and II in different liver disease with hepatocytic membrane expression of HBsAg. Hepatology 5: 1049

Facchetti F, Tardanico R, Bonetti MF, Guerini A, Callea F (1986) HBsAg, HBcAg and Delta-Ag in liver tissue. Simultaneous visualization in a single tissue section by triple immunostaining. Histology and Histopathology 1: 181–185

Furuta S, Kiyosawa K, Nagata A, Akahane Y, Oda M (1975) HBsAg on cell membrane in sympthom free carrier. Lancet ii: 227

Gowans EJ, Burrel CJ (1985) Widespread presence of cytoplasmic HBcAg in hepatitis B infected liver detected by improved immunochemical methods. J Clin Pathol 38: 393–398

Gudat F, Bianchi L (1977a) Evidence for phasic sequence in nuclear HBcAg formation and cell membrane-directed flow of core particles in chronic hepatitis B. Gastroenterology 73: 1194–1197

Gudat F, Bianchi L (1977b) HBsAg: A target antigen on the liver cell? In: Popper H, Bianchi L (eds) Membrane alterations as basis of liver injury. MTP Press, Lancaster, pp 171–178

Hadziyannis S, Gerber MA, Vissoulis C, Popper H (1973) Cytoplasmic hepatitis B antigen in "ground-glass" hepatocytes of carriers. Arch Pathol 96: 327–330

Hodges JR, Millward-Sadler GH, Barbatis C, Wright R (1981) Heterozygous MZ alpha-1-antitrypsin deficiency in adults with chronic active hepatitis and cryptogenic cirrhosis. N Engl J Med 304: 447–560

Hsu SM, Raine L, Fanger H (1981) Use of avidin-biotin-peroxidase complex (ABC) in immunoperoxidase techniques. A comparison between ABC and unlabeled antibody (PAP) procedures. J Histochem Cytochem 29: 577–580

Huang SN, Neurath AR (1979) Immunohistologic demonstration of hepatitis B viral antigens in liver with reference to its significance in liver injury. Lab Invest 40: 1–17

Kamimura T, Ponzetto A, Bonino F, Feinstone SM, Gerin JL, Purcell RH (1983) Cytoplasmic tubular structures in liver of HBsAg Carrier chimpanzees infected with Delta agent and comparison with cytoplasmic structures in non-A, non-B hepatitis. Hepatology 3: 631–637

Kojima T (1982) Immune electron microscopic study of hepatitis B virus associated antigens in hepatocytes. Gastroenterol Jpn 17: 558–575

Kojima T, Desmet VJ (1984) Hepatitis B core antigen (HBcAg) in liver cell plasma membrane: immunoelectron microscopic study. Meeting IASL Berne Sept 3–4 (Abstr) 122

Kojima T, Callea F, Desmyter J, Desmet VJ (1985) Immunoelectron microscopic study of hepatitis Delta antigen (HDAg) in hepatocytes. Hepatology 5: 957

Lock ASF, Lindsay I, Scheuer PJ, Thomas MC (1985) Clinical and histological features of delta infection in chronic hepatitis B virus carriers. J Clin Pathol 38: 530–533

Meyer zum Buschenfelde KH, Hütteroth TH, Arnold W, Hopf U (1979) Immunologic liver injury: The role of hepatitis B viral antigens and liver membrane antigens as targets. In: Popper H, Schaffner F (eds) Progress in liver disease, vol VI. Grune & Stratton, New York, pp 407–424

Mondelli M, Naumov N, Eddlestone ALF (1984) The immunopathogenesis of liver cell damage in chronic hepatitis B virus infection. In: Chisari FV (ed) Advances in hepatitis research. Masson, New York, pp 144–151

Negro F, Chiaberge E, Oliviero S, Hammer M, Berninger M, Canese MG, Bonino F (1984) Hepatitis B virus DNA (HBV-DNA) in anti-HBe positive sera. Liver 4: 177–183

Nowoslawski A, Brzosko WJ, Madalinski K, Krawczynski K (1970) Cellular localization of Australia antigen in the liver of patients with lymphoproliferative disorders. Lancet 1: 494–498

Nowoslawski A, Krawczynski K, Nazarewicz T, Slusarczyk J (1975) Immunopathological aspects of hepatitis type B. Am J Med Sci 270: 229–239

Popper H, Thung SN, Gerber MA, Hadler SC, De Monzon M, Ponzetto A, Anzola E, Rivera D, Mondolfi A, Bracho A, Francis DP, Gerin JL, Maynard JE, Purcell RH (1983) Histologic studies of severe Delta antigen infection in Venezuelan Indians. Hepatology 3: 906–912

Ray MB, Desmet VJ, Bradburne AF, Fevery J, Desmyter J, De Groote J (1976) Differential distribution of hepatitis B surface antigen and hepatitis B core antigen in the liver of hepatitis B patients. Gastroenterology 71: 462–467

Rizzetto M, Canese MG, Aricò S, Crivelli O, Trepo C, Bonino F, Verme G (1977) Immunofluorescent detection of new antigen-antibody system (δ/anti-δ) associated to Hepatitis B virus in liver and serum of HBsAg carriers. Gut 18: 997–1003

Rizzetto M, Verme G, Recchia S, Bonino F, Farci P, Aricò S, Calzia R, Picciotto A, Colombo M, Popper H (1983) Chronic HBsAg hepatitis with intrahepatic expression of Delta antigen. An active and progressive disease unresponsive to immunosuppressive treatment. Ann Intern Med 98: 437–441

Rizzetto M (1983) The Delta agent. Hepatology 3: 729–737

Schweitzer IL, Dunn AEG, Peters RL, Spears RL (1973) Viral hepatitis B in neonats and infants. Am J Med 55: 762–771

Shikata T, Uzawa T, Yoshiwara N, Akatsuka T, Yamazaki S (1974) Staining methods of Australia antigen in paraffin section. Detection of cytoplasmic inclusion bodies. Jpn Exp Med 44: 25–36

Smedile A, Farci P, Verme G, Caredda F, Cargnel A, Caporaso N, Dentico P, Trepo C, Opolon P, Gimson A, Vergani D, Williams R, Rizzetto M (1982) Influence of delta infection on severity of hepatitis B. Lancet 2: 945–947

Tanaka K, Mori W, Suwa S (1981) Victoria blue-nuclear fast red stain for HBsAg antigen detection in paraffin section. Acta Pathol Jpn 31: 93–98

Tardanico R, Zorzi F, Bonetti F, Guerini A, Albertini A, Zorzi M, Rizzetto M, Callea F (1985) Distribution patterns of HBsAg and HBcAg in Delta-Ag positive liver biopsies. Hepatology 5:1048

Trepo C, Vitviski L, Neurath R, Hashimoto N, Schaefer R, Nemoz G, Prince AM (1976) Detection of e antigen by immunofluorescence in cytoplasm of hepatocytes of HBsAg carriers. Lancet 1: 486

Yamada G, Nakane PK (1977) Hepatitis B core and surface antigens in liver tissue: light and electron microscopic localization by the peroxidase-labeled antibody method. Lab Invest 36: 649–659

Yamada G, Feinberg LE, Nakane PK (1978) Hepatitis B cytologic localization of virus antigens and the role of the immune response. Hum Pathol 9: 93

Verme G, Rocca G, Rizzi R, Mollo F, David E, Solcia E, Sessa F (1983) Histopathology of chronic delta hepatitis. In: Verme G, Bonino F, Rizzetto M (eds) Viral hepatitis and delta infection. Liss, New York, pp 169–176

New Diagnostic Techniques: Hepatitis B Virus-DNA in Serum and Liver

F. BONINO, R.M. BRUNETTO, E. CHIABERGE, and F. NEGRO[1]

1 Introduction

Genetic engineering has advanced dramatically in the past few years. Fragments of DNA are snipped from the genome of viruses, prokaryotes or eukaryotes, and joined to other nucleic acid sequences from quite different animals. Transgenic animals are generated in the laboratory so that hidden somewhere along the twisting chain of their DNA in every cell are alien genes injected by the biologist. The product of this remarkable range of manipulations is described as recombinant DNA. The same techniques are now being successfully used to solve a variety of clinical problems and there are no apparent limits to the applications of these methods. The clinician is also going to be involved for the important implications in diagnosis and therapy.

2 Methods

At the base of recombinant DNA technology lies the ability of restriction enzymes to cleave DNA at particular nucleotide sequences and the property of bacterial plasmids and phages to continue their life style after additional sequences of DNA have been incorporated in their genomes. Using these techniques we can break and rejoin DNA molecules at virtually any desired site.

The entire double-stranded genome or fragments of the hepatitis B virus (HBV-DNA) and plasmid DNA can be cleaved using one restriction enzyme that makes staggered cuts and generates complementary single-stranded ends. Fragments are mixed and joined together so that HBV-DNA and plasmid DNA can anneal and recombine into a chimeric plasmid which is used to transform appropriate bacteria. These microorganisms are selected and cloned and viral DNA is purified in many million copies.

The existence of another peculiar enzyme like reverse transcriptase makes it possible to synthesize a duplex DNA from a single-stranded RNA (for example hepatitis delta virus RNA, HDV-RNA) (Denniston et al. 1984). Because HDV-RNA has not a poly (dA) tail, this is added to the 3' end of the nucleic acid by using terminal transferase and the d-ATP precursor. Like other enzyme that synthesize DNA, reverse transcriptase cannot initiate the formation of a polynucleotide chain without a free prim-

---

1 Division of Gastroenterology, S. Giovanni Battista "Molinette" Hospital, Torino,
Corso Bramante 88, 10126 Torino, Italy

Viral Hepatitis, ed. by F. Callea et al.

ing end. Thus a short poly (dT) sequence is added so that it can anneal with the 3' poly (dA) tail, and it is extended by reverse transcriptase which adds deoxynucleotides one at a time directed by complementary base pairing with the HDV-RNA template. The result is a hybrid molecule consisting of single-stranded HDV-RNA base paired with the complementary DNA strand. The hybrid is treated with alkali to remove RNA, which is degraded, while DNA is not affected. The single-stranded DNA copy of viral RNA is converted into a duplex molecule by the enzyme DNA polymerase I of *E. coli*. The final product is a double-stranded DNA copy of HDV-RNA that can be cloned to generate large amounts of synthetic nucleic acid with the same procedure as used for HBV-DNA. Unfortunately, however, recombinant RNA presents some difficulties. RNA molecules are unstable in vitro and reverse transcriptase has the propensity to stop before it has reached the 5' end of the RNA template. In this case the product of the reaction is a transcript that falls short of representing the entire RNA sequence; these disadvantages have thus far hampered the cloning of the entire HDV-RNA. Cloned viral DNA's are labeled with isotopes or biotin and used as diagnostic reagents (probes) in nucleic acid hybridization assays. These methods are based on the property of the double helices of DNA and that of nitrocellulose. Hydrogens bonds between nucleotides of the DNA duplex can be disrupted by heating or alkali and when all of them are broken the two single strands are completely separated. This process, called denaturation or melting, can be easily reversed when temperature and pH return to normal. If complementary sequences of nucleic acid are present in the solution, they can form hybrids by base pairing during this renaturation process, usually called hybridization. Nucleic acid extracted from serum or tissue is easily purified and denaturated. Single-stranded DNA binds specifically to nitrocellulose and it is fixed to the paper by heating. Labeled viral DNA is hybridized to the filter and complementary sequences are identified. The degree of blackening of the film at autoradiography or the enzymatic staining of the filter can be measured quantitatively and is proportional to the amount of viral nucleic acid hybridized to the probe and present in the sample (Bonino et al. 1985b; Berninger et al. 1982). This procedure allows rapid examination of multiple samples and is sensitive and reproducible. The quantity of HBV-DNA detected correlates with the infectivity of sera titered in chimpanzees (Berninger et al. 1982). Fractions of picograms (0.05–0.01 pg) of viral DNA are determined by autoradiography after a 24-h exposure (Bonino et al. 1985a). The minimal amount of viral nucleic acid detected is equivalent to a concentration of 1×10^4 Dane particles. Assuming that one virion corresponds to 10^3 defective HBsAg particles, the estimated sensitivity is comparable to that of the most sensitive radioimmunoassays for HBsAg. The sensitivity is potentially higher in sera with a lower Dane-particle/HBsAg ratio. HBV-DNA sequence can be detected in serum as well as in liver; however, the simple procedures commonly used in serological assays (spot or slot blot hybridization) do not distinguish between free extrachromosomal or integrated forms of viral nucleic acid. The molecular state of HBV-DNA is analyzed by the Southern transfer method in which DNA molecules are fragmented and fractioned by electrophoresis before blotting and hybridization (Brechot et al. 1983). Different forms of extrachromosomal viral DNA can be detected by the Southern technique, including completely double-stranded HBV-DNA (migrating at the 3.2 kilobase position), supercoiled genomes (about 2 kb), relaxed circular genomes (4 kb), partially double-stranded DNA forms (from 2 to 2.8 kb), RNA-DNA hybrids and single-stranded replication intermediates (1.4 kb). The autoradiography appearance of these forms is usually a diffuse smear below the 4 kb position. A hybridization signal near the origin of the lane in regions of the gel corresponding to DNA fragments larger than 4 kb is suggestive of integration of HBV-DNA. However, weak and diffuse autoradiographic bands are difficult to interpret when large quantities of the extrachromosomic DNA are also present. Characterization of these bands requires further analysis after digestion of the nucleic acids with different restriction enzymes. The specificity of nucleic acid hybridization is critically dependent on the purity of the probe and on the stringency of the conditions of hybridization including temperature, ionic strength, and monovalent cationic concentration. The HBV-DNA probe has to be purified and isolated from bacterial and plasmid vector DNA's to avoid unspecific hybridization with *E. coli* or plasma contaminating the samples. Appropriate negative controls should be introduced in each experiment and filters should be rehybridized to a vector lacking the specific DNA insert or to another probe unrelated with HBV-DNA. Parallel samples may be electrophoresed in agarose gels with reference HBV-DNA and then hybridized by the Southern blot technique to establish whether the positive band migrates at a position corresponding to authentic free viral DNA.

Furthermore, methods are also available for measuring the degree of homology between the HBV-DNA probe and the hybridizing nucleic acid. A major disadvantage of hybridization techniques is the use of radioactive probes; however, this problem is now overcome by the introduction of biotin-labeled probes which provide stable and safe reagents (Brigati et al. 1983). The absolute sensitivity of the techniques, using biotinylated probes for detection of HBV-DNA in serum is about 100 times lower that of radioisotopic methods. However, in routine analysis the number of false negative results is less than 3%. The major handicap of the non radioisotopic procedures is that it is impossible to rehybridize the filters because of the permanent enzymatic staining of the paper.

Viral DNA is also measured by means of the endogenous DNA polymerase activity (DNA-P); DNA-P and the concentration of HBV-DNA as detected by molecular hybridization are generally observed to correlate but they do not always maintain a linear relation (Berninger et al. 1982; Bonino et al. 1981; Negro et al. 1984). Various forms of viral DNA are found inside circulating Dane particles including single-stranded, minus-strand DNA, partially double-stranded, or completely double-stranded genomes (Scotto et al. 1985). Thus, under certain conditions of replication, a proportion of Dane particles might contain viral nucleic acid lacking a suitable template for the DNA-P-directed DNA synthesis. Further studies are needed to establish the relation between these HBV-DNA forms and DNA-P activity, and also to analyze the clinical significance of the different hybridization patterns. Parallel assays for viral DNA, Dane particle-associated HBcAg or HBeAg and for HBV-specific DNA polymerase (DNA-P) activity in serum showed the presence of such markers in only a few of the HBV-DNA positive sera (Bonino et al. 1981; Negro et al. 1984; Yokosuka et al. 1985). These findings indicate that the tests performed identify the HB virion but with different levels of sensitivity. These observations suggest that detection of HBV-DNA by nucleic acid hybridization is the "gold" assay for HBV replication. In laboratories, however, where HBV-DNA probes are not available, the best way to measure HBV virions is to run the

DNA-P test using ^{32}P nucleotides and analyzing the reaction products by slab gel electrophoresis and autoradiography (Imazeki et al. 1985). This procedure is not only more sensitive than the conventional DNA-P method, but also as specific as the Southern blot techniques in the detection of HBV-DNA in serum.

Intracellular HBV-DNA can be also detected by in situ hybridization (Negro et al. 1985; Burrel et al. 1982; Blum et al. 1983). This histochemical technique has been shown to stain replication intermediates of the virus and particularly single-stranded forms of viral DNA in the cytoplasm of hepatocytes (Negro et al. 1985; Burrel et al. 1982; Blum et al. 1983). The staining of HBV-DNA was invariably associated with detection of intrahepatic HBcAg even if the intracellular distribution of the antigen and viral-DNA was asymmetrical. These procedures may facilitate the study of the cellular and subcellular distribution of HBV nuclei acid during the different phases of infection and virus synthesis.

3 Clinical Implications

In the course of acute HBV infection, liver disease is generally self-limited and ceases with termination of viral replication. This event is identified by clearance of hepatitis B surface antigen (HBsAg) from serum and seroconversion to the homologous antibody (anti-HBs). Unfortunately, in a proportion of cases, HBV infection becomes chronic. The natural history of chronic HBV infection is one of slow transition from an early phase of active multiplication of the virus to a second phase where HBV exists only in the integrated form in the host's genome. Active viral infection is often associated with liver disease, while HBV integration usually does not result in liver damage representing the typical condition of the asymptomatic carrier of HBsAg (Alberti et al. 1983, Hoofnagle et al. 1981; Realdi et al. 1980). The replicative phase is conventionally identified by presence of the hepatitis B "e" antigen (HBeAg) in serum. The rising of the homologous antibody (anti-HBe) following clearance of HBeAg is assumed to correspond to the inactive phase of HBV infection. Detection of HBV-DNA in serum and liver has changed this concept. Free forms of viral nucleic acid have been found in the serum and liver of the majority of HBeAg positive individuals, but also in a considerable proportion of HBsAg carriers circulating anti-HBe.

In patients with acute type B hepatitis, serum HBV-DNA is usually present during the acute phase of infection and it is cleared before or simultaneously with HBeAg (Bonino et al. 1985b; Krogsgaard et al. 1985). Disappearance of viral DNA is also documented in HBeAg-positive carriers of HBsAg who spontaneously seroconvert to anti-HBe. In a minority of these patients, however, HBV-DNA may circulate for several months beyond clearance of HBeAg (Krogsgaard et al. 1985).

During the period of conversion a discrepancy between the presence of serum HBV-DNA and that of HBeAg is possible. In patients with a prolonged interlude between the active and inactive phase of HBV infection, this discrepancy may be more evident. The viral nucleic acid is in fact a direct measure of virion particles, while HBeAg represents a soluble nucleocapsidic protein of HBV. Thus, detection of HBeAg is dependent on the relative excess of the antigen over the homologous antibody at the time of testing. Another condition of discrepancy between HBV-DNA and HBeAg is the spontaneous reactivation of viral replication, which is a well-described phenomenon in anti-HBe-positive carriers of HBsAg (Krogsgaard et al. 1985; Hoofnagle et al. 1981). A situation where viral DNA and anti-HBe may coexist in serum is also that of the HBsAg carrier coinfected or superinfected with the hepatitis delta virus (HDV). In patients with acute HBV/HDV infection, HBV-DNA is cleared from serum earlier than in patients with HBV infection alone (Krogsgaard et al. 1985). This is due to the inhibitory effect exerted by the defective agent on the synthesis of the helper virus, and it is documented also in carriers of HBsAg with chronic HDV infection (with HDV-RNA in serum and hepatitis delta antigen, HDAg in liver) (Bonino et al. 1985b). These patients are usually positive for anti-HBe and most of them are negative for HBV-DNA; a minority have a small amount of viral nucleic acid in serum. In all these conditions, however, HBV-DNA is detected in serum for a limited period of time. A proportion of sera from anti-HBe-positive carriers of HBsAg without markers of HDV infection may contain HBV-DNA for a long period of follow-up (Bonino et al. 1981; Negro et al. 1984; Yokosuka et al. 1985). A relationship was found between the presence of HBV-DNA in serum and liver disease, since viral DNA was found in 50–70% of anti-HBe-positive carriers with chronic hepatitis, but in none of those with a normal liver (Bonino et al. 1981; Negro et al. 1984; Hadziyannis et al. 1983; Lieberman et al. 1983; Bonino et al. 1986). On the other hand, only 25% of the patients without evidence of HBV replication had liver disease (Negro et al. 1984; Hadziyannis et al. 1983; Lieberman et al. 1983; Bonino et al. 1986). The presence of HBV-DNA in serum of anti-HBe carriers (negative for markers of HDV infection) seems to correlate with an unusual type of intrahepatic assembly of HBcAg. Discrete to large quantities of this antigen are detected predominantly in the cell's cytoplasm opposite the prevalent nuclear localization in HBeAg-positive carriers of HBsAg (Negro et al. 1984; Lieberman et al. 1983; Hadziyannis et al. 1983; Bonino et al. 1986). This atypical anti-HBe/HBV-DNA pattern is also associated with a histological picture of severe chronic hepatitis, whose activity persists unabated through the years leading to cirrhosis in a large proportion of cases (Bonino et al. 1986). One possible interpretation of these results is that HBV-DNA synthesis in the presence of anti-HBe represents a late stage of the natural history of HBV infection, following clearance of HBeAg. Longitudinal studies of HBeAg-positive carriers indicate that this hypothesis may explain only a few cases (Krogsgaard et al. 1985). Seroconversion from HBeAg to anti-HBe is almost invariably followed by remission of liver disease. Rarely, viral DNA persists or reappears in serum of many anti-HBe-positive carriers who had never been found to be HBeAg-positive; viral DNA remained detectable in the serum of these patients for more than 8 years (Bonino et al. 1986). This evidence suggests that HBV replication is an integral component of their serological profile and not an incidental occurrence like the reactivation of the virus. Similar results have been reported by other groups, indicating that the HBV-DNA/anti-HBe syndrome accounts for a large proportion of severe liver disease in HBsAg carriers of Mediterranean and Oriental origin (Hadziyannis et al. 1983; Lieberman et al. 1983; Tur-Kaspa et al. 1984; Chu et al. 1985). The evidence that this atypical HBV-DNA synthesis is more common in males of these areas suggests that it may depend on a genetic predisposition or on unknown environmental factors influencing an early clearance of HBeAg disparate from that of HBcAg from liver and HBV-DNA serum. Wether a delta-like pathogen is responsible for liver disease in these patients remains to be established.

Thus detection of HBV-DNA in serum has many clinical implications: it may be a useful tool for diagnosis and a guide for prognosis. In HBeAg-positive carriers, disappearance of viral nucleic acid from serum generally precedes anti-HBe seroconversion, but unfortunately this event does not preclude chronic infection. A decrease of viral replication in a chronic carrier of HBsAg may indicate either a spontaneous regression of HBV replication preceding an improvement in the clinical picture or the inhibition of HBV synthesis exerted by superinfection of HDV, heralding a deterioration in the liver disease. Finally, persistence of HBV-DNA in serum of long-lasting carriers of anti-HBe (HBsAg-positive and negative for markers of HDV) suggests an unfavorable outcome of chronic hepatitis. The availability of cDNA clones of HDV-RNA allows the application of hybridization techniques also to detection of HDV-RNA; the presence of HDV nucleic acid in serum is a reliable index of active HDV replication (Smedile et al. 1984). These observations indicate the complementary diagnostic value of simultaneous detection of HBV-DNA and HDV markers in HBsAg-positive sera and the poor prognosis of liver disease associated with presence of HBV-DNA and absence of HBeAg in serum. Thus, at present, using simple noninvasive methods, it is possible to determine active replication of HBV and HDV and define whether liver disease in a given carrier of HBsAg is induced by HBV, HDV, or by both viruses. The close association of the presence of viral nucleic acid in serum with progressive virus-induced lived disease indicates that HBV-DNA and HDV-RNA assays may also be used as a guide to prognosis and therapy. The predictive value of these tests can be pictured as that of the weather report provided by the meteorologist (Fig. 1). Patients with a positive test may benefit from the administration of drugs interfering with viral replication (interferons etc.). Quantitative analysis of viral nucleic acid in serum provides the best tool for monitoring the efficacy of these drugs in clinical trials.

Southern hybridization technique has been used to investigate the mechanisms which regulate integration of HBV-DNA, to localize the integration to specific chromosomes and to study the possible existence of preferential sites of viral integration in cellular DNA and hypothetical rearrangements of protoncogenes (Varmus and Summers 1985).

The mechanisms of integration are as yet incompletely defined; in the many tumors analyzed there is no evidence that a unique chromosomal site is used for HBV integration. This appears to occur rather randomly and can be associated with extensive rearrangment of cellular DNA or partial deletion of viral sequences. No correlation between HBV integration and expression of known oncogenes has been found (Varmus and Summers 1985).

The simultaneous detection of complete HBV genomes and replication intermediates in liver indicates active viral replication and it is invariably associated with the presence of viral DNA in serum. The finding of free HBV genomes without replication intermediates suggests spontaneous or drug-induced remission of viral replication (Yokosuka et al. 1985). Positive HBV-DNA hybridization has been found with nuclear acid extracts from kidney, pancreas, skin, sperm, and white blood cells (Brechot et al. 1983; Varmus and Summers 1985). Detection of viral DNA in peripheral blood lymphocytes is intriguing and inviting at the same time (Pontisso et al. 1984; Korba and Gerin 1985). More extensive studies, however, are needed to define the implications of direct invasion of the immune system in the natural history of HBV infection.

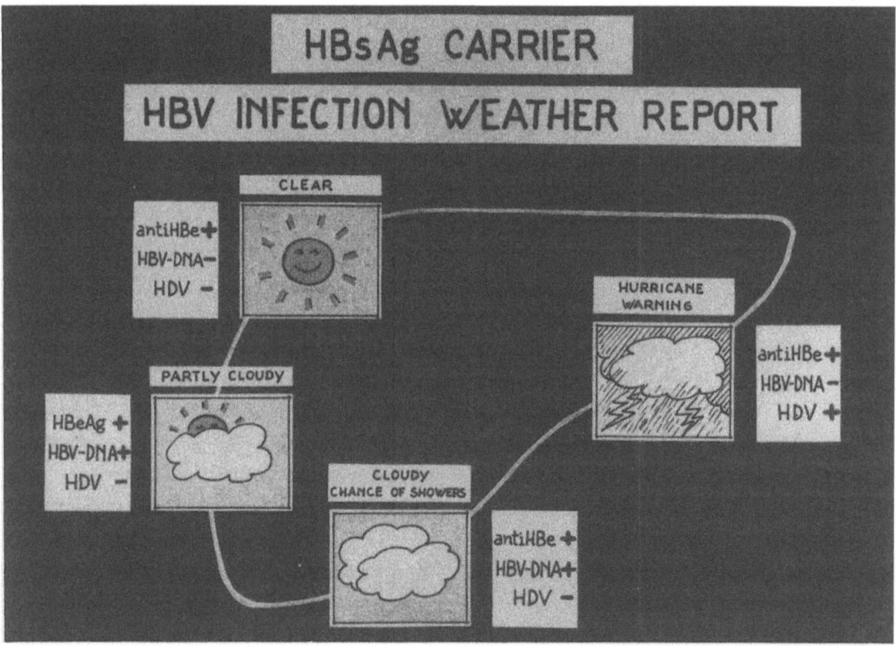

Fig. 1. Prognosis of liver disease in chronic HBsAg carriers. Absence of HBV-DNA and HDV-RNA in serum is a good prognostic sign, being associated with the healthy carrier state. Serum HBV-DNA and HBeAg in absence of HDV marker are indicative of active HBV infection with a good chance of recovery upon anti-HBe seroconversion. Persistence of HBV-DNA in serum of anti-HBe positive carriers is associated with severe and progressive liver disease. The worst outcome is expected in chronic carriers of HBsAg with HDV-RNA in serum as marker of active HDV infection

Thus molecular hybridization represents a powerful tool for research purpose, but it is not without shortcomings when applied in routine analysis. The first of these lies in the results, that differ markedly from the results of conventional techniques. Hybridization signals suggestive of integration have been identified in the livers of patients with chronic hepatitis or primary hepatocellular carcinoma, who were negative not only for HBsAg but also for antibody to HBsAg (anti-HBs) and HBcAg (anti-HBc) (Shafritz 1985). HBV-DNA was detected in serum of chimpanzees with experimental non-A, non-B hepatitis at a time when they were positive for HBsAg, as detected by a monoclonal anti-HBs, but negative by conventional polyclonal assays (Wands et al. 1982). In contrast, other laboratories have reported the absence of HBV-DNA sequences in similar circumstances (Feinstone and Hoofnagle 1984). Therefore, these findings may be interpreted as evidence that HBV may play a pathogenetic role in some cases of non-A, non-B hepatitis and HBsAg-negative tumors or as lack of specificity of the hybridization. Detection of HBV-DNA under unexpected circumstances should be carefully scrutinized before being accepted, but we should also be prepared to admit that the solid ground on which we base our current knowledge may be quickly changed by new discoveries. Unfortunately, however, few studies include appropriate controls, and these additional studies are not always possible because the material obtained from a single needle biopsy is generally insufficient. Thus, at present, the application of molecular hybridization to detection of viral nucleic acid in tissue is very useful in research laboratories, but the clinical implications are limited.

Figus et al. (1984) cloned and sequenced a DNA fragment that hybridized to HBV-DNA and was extracted from the liver of a HBsAg-negative, anti-HBc-positive patient. The sequence appeared to be authentic HBV-DNA integrated in the host genome, but with a mutation within the HBsAg coding sequence hampering the expression of the antigen. Thus we should expect that some individuals who are anti-HBs and anti-HBc positive in absence of HBsAg may harbor HBV-DNA in their liver as the carriers of HBsAg. The extent of this phenomenon and whether it explains also some results in patients without any marker of HBV in serum remains to be explored.

In conclusion, the new techniques provided by recombinant DNA allow not only the study of the mysteries of molecular biology but are becoming familiar in routine analysis and can be used to solve clinical problems. Detection of HBV-DNA and HDV-RNA in serum provides an important diagnostic tool for the hepatologist and a guide for prognosis and therapy.

Acknowledgement: This work was supported by a contract between the Regional Government of Piemonte, Assessorato alla Sanità and the Division of Gastroenterology, S. Giovanni Battista, Molinette Hospital, Torino, Italy.

References

Alberti A, Tremolada F, Fattovich G, Bortolotti F, Realdi G (1983) Virus replication and liver disease in chronic hepatitis B virus infection. Dig Dis Sci 28: 962–966

Berninger M, Hammer M, Hoyer B, Gerin JL (1982) An assay for the detection of the DNA genome of hepatitis B virus in serum. J Med Virol 9: 57–68

Blum EH, Stowring L, Montgomery CK, Haase AP, Vyas GN (1983) Detection of hepatitis B virus DNA in hepatocytes, bile duct epithelium and vacuolar elements by in situ hybridization. Proc Natl Acad Sci USA 80: 6685–6688

Bonino F, Hoyer B, Nelson J, Engle R, Verme G, Gerin JL (1981) Hepatitis B virus DNA in the sera of HBsAg carriers: a marker of active hepatitis B virus replication in the liver. Hepatology 1: 386–391

Bonino F, Chiaberge E, Negro F (1985a) Detection of hepatitis B virus (HBV) DNA by molecular hybridization, clinical significance. In: Koprowski H, Ferrone S, Albertini A (eds) Biotechnology in diagnostics. Elsevier, Amsterdam, pp 163–172

Bonino F, Negro F, Chiaberge E, Brunetto RM, Verme G, Rizzetto M (1985b) Active HBV replication in HBsAg carriers with chronic Delta infection. It J Gastroenterol 17: 235

Bonino F, Rosina F, Rizzetto M, Rizzi R, Chiaberge E, Tardanico R, Callea F, Verme G (1986) Chronic hepatitis in HBsAg carriers with serum HBV-DNA and anti-HBe. Gastroenterology 90: 1268–1273

Brechot C, Dejean A, Tiollais P (1983) Hepatitis B viral DNA sequences in the infected tissues. Prog Clin Biol Res 143: 345–356

Brigati DJ, Myerson D, Leary JJ, Spalholz B, Travis SZ, Fong CKY, Hsiun GD, Ward D (1983) Detection of viral genomes in cultured cells and paraffin-embedded tissue sections using biotin-labeled hybridization probes. Virology 126: 32–50

Burrel CJ, Gowans EJ, Jilbert AR, Lake TR, Marmion BP (1982) Hepatitis B Virus DNA detection by in situ cytohybridization: implications for viral replication strategy and pathogenesis of chronic hepatitis. Hepatology 2: 85–91s

Chu CM, Karaiyannis P, Fowler MJF, Monjardino J, Liaw YF, Thomas HC (1985) Natural history of chronic hepatitis B virus infection in Taiwan: studies of hepatitis B virus DNA in serum. Hepatology 5: 431–434

Denniston KJ, Wells F, Engle R, Hoyer B, Gerin TL (1984) C-DNA cloning of Delta Agent associated RNA and preliminary nucleotide determination. In: Vyas GN, Dienstag JL, Hoofnagle JH (eds) Viral hepatitis and liver disease. Grune & Stratton, New York, pp 696

Feinstone SM, Hoofnagle JH (1984) Non-A, may be-B hepatitis. N Engl J Med 311: 185–189

Figus A, Fung KT, Blum HE, Vyas G, Varmus HE (1984) Definition of a deletion mutant of hepatitis B virus DNA that appears to replicate in the chronically infected liver of a Sardinian patient with B-thalassemia. In: Vyas GN, Dienstag JL, Hoofnagle JH (eds) Viral hepatitis and liver disease. Grune & Stratton, New York, pp 632

Hadziyannis SJ. Lieberman HM, Karvountzis GG, Shafritz DA (1983) Analysis of liver disease, nuclear HBcAg vs anti-HBe positive carriers of Hepatitis B Virus. Hepatology 3: 656–662

Hoofnagle J, Dusheiko GM, Seel LB (1981) Seroconversion from hepatitis B antigen to antibody in chronic type B hepatitis. Ann Intern Med 94: 744–748

Imazeki F, Omata M, Yokosuka O, Matsoyama Y, Ito Y, Okuda K (1985) Analysis of DNA polymerase reaction products for detecting hepatitis B virus in serum–comparison with spot hybridization technique. Hepatology 5: 783–788

Korba BE, Gerin JL (1985) HBV in periferal blood lymphocytes-A comparison between chronically infected patients and animal models. In: Varmus H, Summers J (eds) Molecular Biology of Hepatitis B viruses. Cold Spring Harbor, New York, p 29

Krogsgaard K, Aldershville J, Kryger P, Andersson B, Nielsen JO, Hausson BG and Copenhagen Hepatitis Acute Program (1985) Hepatitis B Virus DNA, HBeAh and Delta infection during the course from acute to chronic Hepatitis B virus infection. Hepatology 5: 778–782

Lieberman HM, La brecque DR, Kew MC, Hadziyannis SJ, Shafritz DA (1983) Detection of Hepatitis B Virus DNA directly in human serum by a simplified molecular hybridization test: comparison to HBeAg/anti-HBa status in HBsAg carriers. Hepatology 3: 285–291

Negro F, Chiaberge E, Oliviero S, Hammer M, Berniner M, Canese MG, Bonino F (1984) Hepatitis B virus (HBV-DNA) in anti-HBe-positive sera. Liver 4: 177–183

Negro F, Berninger M, Chiaberge E, Gugliotta P, Bussolati G, Actis GC, Rizzetto M, Bonino F (1985) Detection of HBV-DNA by in situ hybridization using a biotin-labeled probe. J Med Virol 15: 373–383

Pontisso P, Poon MC, Tiollais P, Brechot C (1984) Detection of hepatitis B virus DNA in mononuclear blood cells. Br Med J 288: 1563–1566

Realdi G, Alberti A, Rugge F, Bortolotti F, Rigoli AM, Tremolada F, Ruol A (1980) Seroconversion from hepatitis B e antigen to anti-HBe in chronic hepatitis B virus infection. Gastroenterology 79: 195–199

Scotto J, Hadchouel M, Wain-Hobson S, Somigo P, Courochè AM, Tiollais P, Brechot C (1985) Hepatitis B virus DNA in Dane particles: evidence for the presence of replicative intermediates. J Infect Dis 151: 610–617

Shafritz DA (1985) Presence of hepatitis B virus deoxyribonucleic acid in human tissues under unexpected circumstances. Gastroenterology 89: 687–690

Smedile A, Rizzetto M, Bonino F, Gerin JL, Hoyer B (1984) Serum Delta associated RNA (DAR) in chronic HBV carriers infected with Delta agent. In: Vyas GN, Dienstag JL, Hoofnagle JH (eds) Viral Hepatitis and liver disease. Grune & Stratton, New York, pp 613

Tur-Kaspa R, Keshet E, Eliakim M, Shouval D (1984) Detection and characterization of hepatitis B virus DNA in serum of HBe antigen-negative HBsAg carriers. J Med Virol 14: 17–26

Varmus H, Summers J (1985) Molecular biology of hepatitis B viruses. Abstracts of papers presented at the 1985 meeting. Cold Spring Harbor, New York

Yokosuka O, Omata M, Imazeki F, Okuda K, Summers J (1985) Changes of hepatitis B virus DNA in liver and serum caused by recombinant leukocyte interferon treatment: analysis of intrahepatic replicative hepatitis B virus DNA. Hepatology 5: 728–734

Wands JR, Lieberman HM, Muchmore E, Isselbacher K, Shafritz OA (1982) Detection and transmission in chimpanzees of hepatitis B virus-related agents formerly designated "nonA, nonB" hepatitis. Proc Natl Acad Sci USA 79: 7552–7556

Lessons from the Pathology of Viral Hepatitis in Animal Models

H. POPPER[1]

1 Introduction

The histogenesis of the various morphologic features in the different types of human viral hepatitis is not established, nor are definite criteria in the histologic distinction agreed upon. Moreover, the mechanism of transition to hepatocellular carcinoma (HCC) is not clarified, including molecular pathobiologic changes. Animal models of viral hepatitis may contribute to the understanding of these problems. The following descriptions are based on histologic material provided by, or studies in cooperation with, H.J. Alter, D.W. Bradley, H.P. Dienes, J.L. Dienstag, S.M. Feinstone, M.A. Gerber, J.L. Gerin, S.C. Hadler, P.L. Marion, A. Ponzetto, R.H. Purcell, M. Rizzetto, W.S. Robinson, D.A. Shafritz, B.C. Tennant, and S.N. Thung. Two types of animal model can be distinguished. One results from experimental inoculation of laboratory animals for such purposes as to (a) characterize the viruses and their immunogenic potencies, particularly when virus culture in cells has not succeeded, (b) prove the infectiosity of such material, e.g., to identify hepatitis non-A, non-B (NANB), (c) determine the safety of vaccines, or effects of therapeutic agents, (d) provide material for vaccines, and (e) study the co- or superinfection with two of the viral agents. The other type entails the investigation of spontaneous infections in both domestic and wild animals.

The material made available for histologic study, performed initially without knowledge of the experimental history, was in general well identified by a study of the serum biochemically for liver injury, as well as serologically and immunologically for viral infection, and, where applicable, liver and serum for the status of the viral DNA by hybridization techniques. The observations entail three aspects, treated in the following sections: the expression of various types of viral hepatitis in experimentally infected chimpanzees and marmosets, the lesions produced by Hepadna viruses in wild and laboratory infected animals, and alterations from experimental infection with two viruses.

2 The Expression of Various Types of Viral Hepatitis in Experimentally Infected Chimpanzees and Marmosets

Particularly in chimpanzees, the correlation between hepatocytic injury and the elevation of the serum activities of enzymes such as alanine aminotransferases is very good, regardless of type of the virus (Popper et al. 1980; Popper 1983).

---

1 The Stratton Laboratory for the Study of Liver Diseases, Mount Sinai School of Medicine, University of New York, One Gustave Levy Place, New York 10029, USA

Viral Hepatitis, ed. by F. Callea et al.
© Springer-Verlag Berlin Heidelberg 1986

In general, necroinflammation in chimpanzees is less severe than in man, and massive necrosis rarely occurs.

A panlobular hepatitis in marmosets infected by hepatitis A-virus-containing human material was the first successful transmission of any human viral hepatitis to animals (Deinhardt et al. 1967; Holmes et al. 1971). Infectious material causes in chimpanzees an acute, eventually completely regressing, hepatitis. It is characterized by severe portal and periportal inflammation, with focal destruction of periportal hepatocytes, but absence of inflammation from the perivenous zone 3 (Popper et al. 1980; Dienstag et al. 1975, 1976). Immunohistochemically, however, hepatitis A antigen can be demonstrated throughout the lobule (Boggs et al. 1970). In man, particularly in children, there is a similar periportal accentuation of necroinflammation. If severe, as in adults, the necroinflammation proceeds to zone 3 (Abe et al. 1982; Teixeira et al. 1982).

Hepatitis B virus material does not infect marmosets, but produces in chimpanzees, after longer incubation period than that of hepatitis A, a panlobular hepatitis with inflammation involving also the hepatic vein tributaries (Abe et al. 1982). It is characterized by an abundance of lymphocytes in close contact with hepatocytes, both normal and altered ones, in agreement with the postulated lymphocytotoxicity characteristic of this infection (Gudat et al. 1975). In contrast to acute hepatitis B in man, however, surface antigen is diffusely distributed around the hepatocytic membranes (Baker et al. 1973). This suggests a lower intensity of the lymphocytic attack in chimpanzees and is in keeping with less severe inflammation than often seen in man. Only rarely is bridging necrosis observed in the chimpanzee. The disease subsides more slowly than hepatitis A, and a carrier state may exist for many years. In contrast to most human HBsAg carriers, evidence of considerable viral replication persists in the chimpanzees, reflected in high DNA polymerase and e antigen in serum. Ground-glass cells are common, which give distinct orcein reaction of Shikata or stain with Victoria blue (Tanaka et al. 1981). Immunoperoxidase and fluorescence reactions of hepatocytes for surface, and also for core, hepatitis B antigen are positive (Thung et al. 1981). These carrier chimpanzees show histologically no significant lesion or mild chronic persistent hepatitis, with only rare evidence of spread of portal inflammation into periportal parenchyma. Characteristically, the hepatocytic nuclei are normal, and integration of viral DNA sequences into host DNA is not noted (Shouval et al. 1980), in contrast to some human HBsAg carriers. So far, only one chimpanzee with chronic active hepatitis has been observed (Shafritz, personal communication). The lymphocytic predominance in the parenchyma seems to be also characteristic of most cases of human hepatitis B.

The existence of hepatitis non-A, non-B (NANB) has been established by transmission of infectious material from human acute and chronic hepatitis and carriers to chimpanzees and by further transmission to additional chimpanzees (Alter et al. 1978; Tabor et al. 1978). The earlier stages of chimpanzee NANB hepatitis are characterized by increase of sinusoidal cells, including lymphocytes which, however, remain within the sinusoids. This is associated with varying degrees of portal inflammation, which, however, does not spread into the surrounding parenchyma. In many chimpanzees this is followed by a stage characterized by microvesicular steatosis and eosinophilic granulation of the hepatocytic cytoplasm, proceeding to conspicuous acidophilic bodies, while inflammatory cells are sparse in the parenchyma but numerous in the portal tracts (Popper et al. 1980). These portal lymphocyte aggregates surround mildly altered bile ducts. During this stage, aminotransferase activities rise, but not as steeply as in most chimpanzees with hepatitis A or B. This stage is followed in about half of the chimpanzees by a chronic lesion, with occasional and transient moderate rises in aminotransferase activity. Besides irregular portal inflammation corresponding to chronic persisting hepatitis in man, focal necroses in the parenchyma, with acidophilic bodies, are transiently observed. These lesions have been encountered up to 3 years after the initial infection (Bradley et al. 1982).

In analogy with similar lesions in man, hepatitis NANB in chimpanzees is a protracted disorder sometimes with recurrences, but of lesser activity than the other forms of viral hepatitis. The histologic picture suggests cytotoxicity, but not induced by attack by lymphocytes (Dienes et al. 1982), though they may be numerous in sinusoids (Bamber et al. 1981). In all stages, electron microscopically two types of lesion have been described in chimpanzees (Shimizu et al. 1979); one, nuclear particles of non-viral character , and the other, cytoplasmic undulating tubules. In the chronic stages only the latter was found. However, the significance of these features is not established (Schaff et al. 1984). Transmission of infectious NANB material to marmosets produces in at least some of them a transient lesion similar to that in chimpanzees (Feinstone et al. 1981). In preliminary studies with R.H. Purcell on material from human epidemics in India, which did not cause chronic hepatitis and are associated with transmission resembling that in hepatitis A (Khuroo 1980; Balayan et al. 1982), large transient focal necroses have been observed both in chimpanzees and marmosets. Animal experiments thus also suggest more than one type of NANB viral hepatitis, and the possibility that NANB is a variant of hepatitis type B without expression of markers is not excluded (Wands et al. 1982).

3 Lesions Produced by Hepadna Viruses in Wild and Laboratory Infected Animals

Hepadna viruses represent a group of viruses which include besides HBV viruses with considerable similarity to HBV which do not, however, infect man, and the animals susceptible to Hepadna viruses cannot be infected by HBV. The DNA and the antigens have great homology to HBV-DNA and the respective antigens. The woodchuck (*Marmota monax*) hepatitis virus (WHV) was the first described (Snyder et al. 1982; Summers 1981) and shows the greatest homology to HBV. The initial observations concerned caught wild animals in which acute appearing and chronic hepatitis, as well as HCC, were found. In Pennsylvania at least, approximately 40% of the animals were infected, which was not necessarily true of other areas. At least 25% of infected wild woodchucks developed HCC (Robinson et al. 1984). The acute hepatitis shows manifestation similar to the human hepatitis type B, including in the parenchyma focal necrosis, predominance of lymphocytes, acidophilic bodies, and variations of hepatocytes, as well as significant portal inflammation. In contrast to its human counterpart, plasma cells are abundant and hepatocellular nodules are noted even in acute-appearing disease. Chronic hepatitis is similar to human persistent or active hepatitis. In both the acute-appearing and the chronic woodchuck hepatitis, the cytoplasm of isolated hepatocytes shows inclusions, stained by Shikata's orcein stain or by Victoria blue, corresponding to human ground-glass cells (Popper et al. 1981). The HCC exibits distinct transitions to hyperplastic zones with hepatocytes in two-cell-thick plates, and further to normal parenchyma, corresponding to "nodules in nodules" (Popper 1977). The carcinoma cells express conspicuous variations similar to man, from typical trabecular to anaplastic and even cholangiolar carcinoma.

Thus the HCC resembles that in man in histologic appearance and in the integration of viral into chromosomal DNA, both in the tumor and in the surrounding parenchyma. However, the integrated WHV-DNA and the flanking sequences are in normal arrangement in chronic hepatitis except for some deletion in the WHV-DNA, while both are disorganized in HCC (Rogler and Summers 1984), The woodchuck HCC differs from the human by its development in acute-appearing hepatitis, by the common absence of cirrhosis, by the presence of many hematopoietic cells, and by not only e antigen, but also WHV-DNA and polymerase in the serum as indication of active viral replication, which is rare in human HCC (Popper et al. 1981).

In recent, so far unpublished experiments with J.L. Gerin, B.C. Tennant et al., laboratory-infected woodchucks were examined which showed similar features of acute, sometimes quite florid hepatitis, and a WHV surface antigen carriers state with appearance of Victoria blue-positive hepatocytes 1 year after the infection. In four out of four woodchucks infected shortly after birth, in which such a WHV carrier state with mild inflammatory changes but Victoria blue-positive cells developed, hepatocytic nodules and subsequently HCC developed within a year and 1/4. These tumors were associated with an active hepatitis. Moreover, in several woodchucks infected as adults, HCC set in, also associated with a reactivation of the hepatitis and Victoria blue-positive hepatocytes. Again, transition to nodules could be demonstrated.

In Beechey ground squirrels in California, but again, not in other regions, a Hepadna virus (GSBH) was isolated, associated with hepatitis in some squirrels and also Victoria blue-positive hepatocytes (Marion et al. 1983). So far several hepatocellular carcinomas have been observed in association with GSBH (Marion et al. 1986).

In ducks in China, both chronic hepatitis and hepatocellular carcinoma have been found associated with a Hepadna virus (DHBV). This virus shows less homology to HBV than the other Hepadna viruses, but has served as a valuable model to study the replication pattern of the entire group. However, similar hepatitis has been observed in the absence of the virus. Recently, the DNA has been found integrated in the host DNA in HCC (Yokosuka et al. 1985). Histologically, the HCC somewhat differs from the human variety, but less so than the chronic hepatitis, in which Victoria blue-positive hepatocytes may be abundant and often in clusters. Domestic ducks, particularly Pekin ducks, may be infected with the same virus, apparently by maternal transmission but without producing histological alterations (O'Connell et al. 1983). Injection, however, of the virus into the egg or into the newly hatched duckling results in a characteristic hepatitis with both lobular and portal manifestations (Marion et al. 1984). This may be the cheapest way to produce viral hepatitis experimentally.

The Hepadna viruses thus present laboratory models not only for molecular biologic study and for investigations of both vaccination and antiviral therapy, but also on a histologic level to explore the evolution of hepatitis, particularly chronic and the transition to hepatocellular nodules and HCC, as well as, foremost, to prove the carcinogenic potency of this group of viruses and in analogy of HBV.

4 Alterations from Experimental Infection with Two Viruses

Infection of HBsAg carrier chimpanzees with hepatitis A-containing material produces a lesion with all the histological characteristics of chimpanzees hepatitis A infection, but of considerably more severe degree, for instance, including injury to bile ducts (Dienes et al. 1981). These observations are in keeping with human experiences of transient depression of HBV replication during hepatitis A superinfection. Similarly, superinfection of HBV carrier chimpanzees with NANB infectious material results in a far more severe expression of the previously described NANB lesion, including confluent necrosis with collapse, associated with many acidophilic bodies in the surrounding parenchyma. The HBsAg serum level transiently declines (Dienes et al. 1981).

The most impressive example is the superinfection of chimpanzees HBsAg carriers by delta (D) agent-containing material (Rizzetto et al. 1980). Most of the chimpanzees develop a very severe hepatitis characterized by conspicuous swelling of hepatocytes with cytoplasmic alterations which include, besides some small-droplet steatosis, irregular clumping. The hepatocytes are surrounded by many macrophages with PAS-positive, diastase-resistant granules and by relatively few lymphocytes. The portal tracts contain many inflammatory cells, some of which extend into the surrounding parenchyma in the sense of a piecemeal necrosis. During this stage, the previously present Victoria blue-positive hepatocytes have disappeared and much lipofuscin is seen in macrophages (Dienes et al. 1981), associated with a transient suppression of HBV replication. Weekly serial biopsies indicate resolution of the lesion within 2 or 3 weeks and, in some chimpanzees, conspicuous regeneration of the hepatocytes. After several weeks, Victoria blue-positive hepatocytes are noted again. In a few chimpanzees, the transient lesion has a great histological resemblance to chimpanzee hepatitis NANB. The similarity between D- and NANB-induced hepatitis, both of which, on light microscopy, show conspicuous cytotoxic changes, is also in keeping with electron microscopic observations (Kamimura et al. 1983). Only in one chimpanze, which had anti-e antibodies at the time of the superinfection, has a chronic D hepatitis been reported (Govindarajan and Fields 1984). Co-infection by HBV and D agents of a few chimpanzees has produced irregular and mild changes, in contrast to the superinfection, which causes the most severe type of chimpanzee viral hepatitis seen so far (Dr. Ponzetto, personal communication).

Recently, transmission of D agent-containing material from chimpanzees to WHV-carrier woodchucks with essentially normal liver except for Victoria blue-positive hepatocytes resulted in an acute hepatitis with destruction of Victoria blue-positive hepatocytes. This was associated with expression of D agent and suppression of WHV replication (Ponzetto et al. 1984). These observations indicate that WHV can provide, similarly to HBV, surface antigen for the D virus. Of further interest is that after subsidence of the D hepatitis in the woodchuck, another bout of acute hepatitis developed with the characteristic histologic and virologic features of a WHV hepatitis, thus representing a rebound.

The experience with superinfection indicates that the histologic expression characteristic for a type of chimpanzee viral hepatitis, for instance, type A or NANB, breeds through in superinfections. Moreover, the observation that superinfection, including with the D agents, not only produces a more severe form of hepatitis, but also suppresses HBV replication, has potential applications to human pathology. While originally progression of chronic hepatitis was believed to develop by relentless extension of piecemeal necrosis, now, acute episodes of localized necroinflammation in the sense of a subacute hepatic necrosis are incriminated in the progression (Popper 1983b). These episodes may lead either to death or cirrhosis and possibly also, as a promotion, to HCC, the latter suggested by the observation in woodchucks in which the carcinogenesis is seemingly accelerated. The acute episodes in human hepatitis type B, which may set in after prolonged periods of clinical, histological, and virological quiescence (Davis and Hoofnagle 1985), may result from flare-ups of HBV infection, for instance from an altered immune status. Alternatively, they may reflect superinfection with another virus when HBV replication is reduced. These considerations may direct therapeutic strategies.

5 Conclusions

The morphologic study of animal models of viral hepatitis has provided, in addition to support of virologic, molecular biologic, and therapeutic investigations, lessons as to (a) the distinction of the histological patterns of the different types, (b) pathogenesis, including carcinogenicity, and (c) evolution of chronic hepatitis, which seems to be accelerated in animals. Since it has been difficult to document the evolution, particularly of hepatitis B and NANB, in man over years and decades and many riddles still persist, the study of animal models is bound to continue.

References

Abe H, Beninger PR, Ihejiri N, Setoyama H, Saba M, Tanikawa K (1982) Light microscopic findings of liver biopsy specimens from patients with hepatitis type A and comparison with type B. Gastroenterology 82: 938–947

Alter HJ, Holland PV, Purcell RH, Popper H (1978) Transmissible agent in non-A, non-B hepatitis. Lancet 1: 459–463

Baker LF, Chisari FV, McGrath PP, Dalgard DW, Kirchstein RL, Almeida JD, Edgington TS, Sharp DG, Peterson MR (1973) Transmission of type B viral hepatitis to chimpanzees. J Infect Dis 127: 648–662

Balayan MS, Andjaparidze AG, Savinskaya SS (1982) Evidence for a causative agent of human non-A, non-B hepatitis transmitted via fecal-oral route. Hepatitis Sci Memoranda 4: 51–52

Bamber M, Murray AK, Weller IVD, Morelli A, Scheuer PJ, Thomas HC, Sherlock S (1981) Clinical and histologic features of a group of patients with sporadic non-A, non-B hepatitis. J Clin Pathol 34: 1175–1180

Bradley DW, Maynard JE, Krawczynski KZ, Popper H, Cook EH, Gravelle CR, Ebert JW (1982) Non-A, non-B hepatitis in chimpanzees infected with a factor VIII agent: Evidence of persistent hepatic disease. In: Szmuness W, AlterHJ, Maynard JE (eds) Viral hepatitis: 1981 symposium. The Franklin Inst Press, Philadelphia, pp 319–329

Boggs JD, Melnick JL, Conrad MD, Felsher BF (1970) Viral hepatitis: clinical and tissue culture studies. J Am Med Assoc 214: 1041–1046

Davis GL, Hoofnagle JH (1985) Reactivation of chronic hepatitis B virus infection presenting as acute viral hepatitis. Ann Intern Med 102: 762–765

Deinhardt F, Holmes AW, Capps RB, Popper H (1967) Studies on the transmission of human viral hepatitis to marmoset monkeys. 1. Transmission of disease, serial passages and description of liver lesions. J Exp Med 125: 673–688

Dienes HP, Purcell RH, Popper H, Bonino F, Ponzetto A (1981) Simultaneous infection of chimpanzees with more than one hepatitis virus. Hepatology 1: 506

Dienes HP, Popper H, Arnold W, Lobeck H (1982) Histologic observations in human hepatitis non-A, non-B. Hepatology 2: 562–571

Dienstag JL, Feinstone SM, Purcell RH, Hoofnagle JH, Barker LF, London WT, Popper H, Peterson JM, Kapikian AZ (1975) Experimental infection of chimpanzees with hepatitis A virus. J Infect Dis 132: 532–545

Dienstag JL, Popper H, Purcell RH (1976) The pathology of viral hepatitis types A and B in chimpanzees. A comparison. Am J Pathol 85: 131–148

Feinstone SM, Alter HJ, Dienes HP, Shimizu U, Popper H, Blackmore D, Sly D, London WT, Purcell RH (1981) Non-A, non-B hepatitis in chimpanzees and marmosets. J Infect Dis 144: 588–598

Govindarajan S, Fields HA (1984) Chronic delta infection in a chimpanzee with apparent remission and exacerbation–a morphological study. In: Vyas GN, Dienstag JL, Hoofnagle JH (eds) Viral hepatitis and liver disease. Grune & Stratton, New York, pp 614

Gudat F, Bianchi L, Sonnabend W, Thiel G, Ainishaenslin W, Stalder GA (1975) Pattern of core and surface expression in liver tissue reflects state of specific immune response in hepatitis B. Lab Invest 32: 1–9

Holmes AW, Wolfe L, Deinhardt F, Conrad ME (1971) Transmission of human hepatitis to marmosets. Further coded studies. J Infect Dis 124: 520–521

Kamimura T, Ponzetto A, Bonino F, Feinstone SM, Gerin TL, Purcell RM (1983) Cytoplasmic tubular structures in liver of HBsAg carrier chimpanzees infected with delta agent and comparison with cytoplasmic structures in non-A, non-B hepatitis. Hepatology 3: 631–637

Khuroo MS (1980) Study of an epidemic on non-A, non-B hepatitis. Am J Med 68: 818–824

Marion PL, Knight SS, Salazar FH, Popper H, Robinson WS (1983) Ground squirrel hepatitis virus infection. Hepatology 3: 519–527

Marion PL, Knight SS, Ho B-K, Guo Y-Y, Robinson WS, Popper H (1984) Liver diseases associated with duck hepatitis B virus infection of domestic ducks. Proc Natl Acad Sci USA 81: 898–902

Marion PL, Van Davelaar MJ, Knight SS, Salazar FH, Garcia G, Popper H, Robinson WS (1986) Hepatocellular carcinoma in ground squirrels persistently infected with ground squirrel hepatitis virus. Proc Natl Acad Sci USA 83: 4543–4546

O'Connell AP, Urban MK, London WT (1983) Naturally occurring infection of Pekin duck embryos by duck hepatitis B virus. Proc Natl Acad Sci USA 80: 1703–1706

Ponzetto A, Cote PJ, Popper H, Hoyer BH, London WT, Fort EC, Bonino F, Purcell RH, Gerin JL (1984) Transmission of the hepatitis B virus associated delta agent to the eastern woodchuck. Proc Natl Acad Sci USA 81: 2208–2212

Popper H (1977) Pathologic aspects of cirrhosis. A review. Am J Pathol 87: 228–264

Popper H, Dienstag JL, Feinstone SM, Alter HJ, Purcell RH (1980) The pathology of viral hepatitis in chimpanzees. Virchows Arch A Pathol Anat Histol 387: 91–106

Popper H, Shih JW-K, Gerin JL, Wong DC, Hoyer BH, London WT, Sly DL, Purcell RH (1981) Woodchuck hepatitis and hepatocellular carcinomas: Correlation of histologic with virologic observations. Hepatology 1: 91–98

Popper H (1983) Pathology of viral hepatitis. In: Overby L, Deinhardt F, Deinhardt J (eds) Viral hepatitis. 2nd Int Max von Pettenkofer Symposium. Dekker, New York, pp 11–18

Popper H (1983b) Changing concepts of the evolution of chronic hepatitis and role of piecemeal necrosis. Hepatology 3: 758–762

Rizzetto M, Canese MG, Gerin JL, London WT, Sly DL, Purcell DH (1980) Transmission of the hepatitis B virus-associated delta antigen to chimpanzees. J Infect Dis 141: 590–602

Rogler CE, Summers J (1984) Cloning and structural analysis of integrated woodchuck hepatitis virus sequences from a chronically infected liver. J Virol 50: 832–837

Robinson WS, Marion PL, Miller RH (1984) The Hepadna viruses of animals. Semin Liver Dis 4: 347–360

Schaff Z, Tabor E, Jackson DR, Gerety RJ (1984) Ultrastructural alterations in serial liver biopsy specimens from chimpanzees experimentally infected with a human non-A, non-B hepatitis agent. Virchows Arch B Cell Pathol 45: 301–312

Shimizu YK, Feinstone SM, Purcell RH (1979) Non-A, non-B hepatitis: ultrastructural evidence for two agents in experimentally infected chimpanzees. Science 205: 197–200

Shouval D, Chakraborty PR, Ruis-Opazo N, Baum S, Spigland I, Muchmore E, Gerber MA, Thung SN, Popper H, Shafritz DA (1980) Chronic hepatitis in chimpanzees carriers of hepatitis B virus: morphologic, immunologic and viral DNA studies. Proc Natl Acad Sci USA 77: 6147–6151

Snyder RL, Tyler G, Summers J (1982) Chronic hepatitis and hepatocellular carcinoma associated with woodchuck hepatitis virus. Am J Pathol 107: 422–425

Summers J (1981) Three recently described animal virus models for human hepatitis B virus. Hepatology 1: 179–183

Tabor E, Gerety RJ, Drucker JA, Seef LB, Hoofnagle HJ, Jackson DR, April M, Baker LF, Pineda-Tamondong G (1978) Transmission of non-A, non-B hepatitis from man to chimpanzee. Lancet 1: 463–466

Tanaka K, Mori W, Suwa K (1981) Victoria blue-nuclear fast red stain for HBs antigen detection in paraffin section. Acta Pathol Jpn 31: 93–98

Teixeira MR Jr, Weller IVD, Murray A, Bamber M, Thomas HC, Sherlock S, Scheuer PJ (1982) The pathology of hepatitis A in man. Liver 2: 53–60

Thung SN, Gerber MA, Purcell RH, London WT, Mihalik KB, Popper H (1981) Animal model of human disease: chimpanzee carriers of hepatitis B virus. Am J Pathol 105: 328–332

Wands JR, Lieberman HM, Muchmore E, Isselbacher K, Shafritz DA (1982) Detection and transmission in chimpanzees of hepatitis B virus-related agents formerly designated "non-A, non-B" hepatitis. Proc Natl Acad Sci USA 79: 7552–7556

Yokosuka O, Omata M, Zhou Y-Z, Imazeki F, Okuda K (1985) Duck hepatitis B virus DNA in liver and serum of Chinese ducks: Integration of viral DNA in a hepatocellular carcinoma. Proc Natl Acad Sci USA 82: 5180–5184

A Review of the Efficacy of Adenine Arabinoside and Lymphoblastoid Interferon in the Royal Free Hospital Studies of Hepatitis B Virus Carrier Treatment: Identification of Factors Influencing Response Rates

H.C. THOMAS, L.J. SCULLY, A.M.L. LEVER, I. YAP, and M. PIGNATELLI[1]

1 Introduction

Many anti-viral agents have been tried in the treatment of chronic HBV infection (Pollard et al. 1978; Weller et al. 1982, 1983; Greenberg et al. 1976; Lok et al. 1984a; Smith et al. 1983). Only adenine arabinoside in both its native and monophosphate forms and the alpha interferons have been evaluated to a level where comments on clinical usefulness can be made.

2 Adenine Arabinoside and Its Monophosphate

In 1977 adenine arabinoside was evaluated in a randomised controlled trial and 40% of patients treated were found to undergo HBeAg/Ab seroconversion (Table 1) (Bassendine et al. 1981). This was followed by a reduction in the inflammatory activity in the liver. No such changes were observed in the control group derived from the same population of hepatitis B virus carriers. Because of the need to give adenine arabinoside by continuous intravenous infusion, the duration of treatment had to be limited, and when the highly water-soluble monophosphate derivative became available and bolus intramuscular therapy became possible, controlled trials were started with this compound (Hoofnagle et al. 1984; Weller et al. 1985).

Studies demonstrated that twice-daily injections were adequate to maintain inhibition of virus replication and the best results were obtained with a 5-day induction course at a dosage of 10 mg/kg per day followed by a maintenance course at half this dosage level for a further 23 days (Weller et al. 1982). This course avoided the complications of peripheral neuropathy which were subsequently reported from America (Hoofnagle et al. 1984; Sacks et al. 1982). These neurological problems are related to the cumulative total dose (Lok et al. 1984b). A randomised controlled trial was undertaken at the Royal Free Hospital and 40% of patients receiving this 1-month course of adenine arabinoside underwent HBe/anti-HBe conversion within 18 months of treatment, whereas no such changes occurred in the control group (Weller et al. 1985). In both this randomised controlled study and in the study with adenine arabinoside, the increased rate of HBeAg/Ab seroconversion rates seen in the treated patients was signi-

---

1 Academic Department of Medicine, Royal Free Hospital and School of Medicine, Pond Street, Hampstead, London NW3 2QG, United Kingdom

Viral Hepatitis, ed. by F. Callea et al.
© Springer-Verlag Berlin Heidelberg 1986

Table 1. Results of randomised trials of antiviral therapy of chronic hepatitis B infection

Response to treatment

Author	No (%) treatment	ARA-A (%)	ARA-AMP (%)	Lymphoblastoid IFN (%)	Recombinant IFN (%)	Steroid + ARA-AMP (%)
Bassendine et al. (1981)	0/ 6 (0%)	3/ 7 (42%)				
Hoofnagle (1982)	2/10 (20%)		2/10 (20%)			
Weller et al. (1985)	0/14 (0%)		6/15 (40%)			
Lok (1985)			4/15 (27%) (4 weeks) 0/14 (0%) (8 weeks)	5/16 (31%)		
Perillo et al. (1985)	1/17 (6%)		0/11 (4 weeks) 1/ 7 (8 weeks)			
Dusheiko (1985)	0/11 (0%)				6/14 (43%)	
Yokosuka et al. (1985)	2/10 (20%)	1/10 (10%)				6/9 (67%)
Total	5/68 (7%)	4/17 (23%)	13/72 (18%)	5/16 (31%)	6/14 (43%)	6/9 (67%)

ficantly greater than that seen in the control group. In addition, these seroconversion rates were at least twice the highest levels of spontaneous seroconversion reported in the literature (Realdi et al. 1980; Viola et al. 1981; Liaw et al. 1983). These data were confirmed in a second trial in which a 1-month course of adenine arabinoside was compared with a 7-8-week course of the drug (Lok et al. 1986). The longer-duration therapy often led to symptoms of peripheral neuropathy and the seroconversion rates were worse than those seen with the shorter course of treatment. It was proposed that this poor result with the longer course of adenine arabinoside monophosphate stemmed from the immunosuppressive properties of the drug which prevented recovery of the host immune response necessary for lysis of the residual infected hepatocytes. The results with a month's course of adenine arabinoside monophosphate were encouraging, and when second courses of the drug were used, seroconversion rates of 60–70% were reported (Trepo et al. 1984). In contrast, two American groups (Hoofnagle et al. 1984; Perillo et al. 1985) reported no significant change in seroconversion rates (HBeAg/Ab) when compared to controls. These variable results from different areas of the world led us to consider the factors which might be influencing response in these different groups.

2.1 Factors Influencing Response to Adenine Arabinoside Monophosphate

Data from 48 patients were available for evaluation (Novick et al. 1984). All these patients had been treated within the randomised controlled trials conducted at the Royal Free Hospital (Weller et al. 1985; Lok et al. 1986). It soon became apparent that the response rate in patients coming from Mediterranean countries was of the order of 60–70%, comparable to those seen by Trepo et al. (1984), and, in marked contrast, no responses were seen in 24 patients native to London (Table 2). The majority of these patients were homosexual carriers (Novick et al. 1984).

An analysis of the additional factors determining response and non-response (Novick et al. 1984) confirmed the observation of Scullard et al. (1981) that those patients with the highest transaminases and with the most active liver biopsies tended to respond to this form of treatment, whereas those with low transaminases and chronic persistent or minimal hepatitis did not respond.

Close examination of the sequence of events during adenine arabinoside monophosphate treatment reveals that the transaminases rise on stopping treatment (Fig. 1). We suspect that adenine arabinoside inhibits HBV replication, by affecting the efficiency of transcription of the viral genome, and in addition, because of its effect on host DNA synthesis, is immunosuppressive. Thus, although the drug effectively inhibits viral replication, long-term effects will only be seen if the host immune response is able to recover and to destroy the residual virus-infected cells. This occurs after cessation of treatment and is marked by the rise in transaminase. Longer periods of adenine arabinoside treatment stop this immune recovery from occurring and prevent long-term effects (Lok et al. 1986). The secondary immunodeficiency found in homosexual patients may also prevent this immune recovery (Novick et al. 1986; Reginstein et al. 1983).

During these studies the prevalence of HTLV III infection in this population was less than 5% (personal observation) and it seems that other factors causing immunode-

Table 2. Response rates (loss of HBeAg and HBV-DNA from the sera) of different patient groups treated in randomised trials at the Royal Free Hospital

Response rates:

Patient group	Treatment ARA-AMP	IFN
Heterosexual males		
Nothern European	7/10	4/ 6
Others	3/12	3/ 5
Heterosexual females		
Nothern European	–	1/ 2
Others	–	0/ 7[b]
Homosexual males		
Nothern European	0/24[a]	12/25[a]
Others	–	0/ 1

[a] $p < 0.05$
[b] Of 8 Chinese (2M; 6F) treated with interferon, none Responded

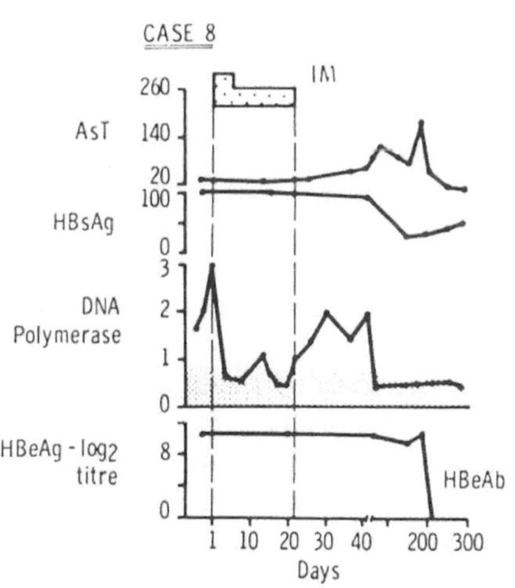

Fig. 1. Treatment with ARA-AMP. During treatment HBV-DNA polymerase activity falls, but rise when ARA-AMP is stopped. The rise in AST indicates lysis of virus infected hepatocytes and the seroconversion from HBeAg to anti-HBe positivity occurs after treatment is completed

ficiency were operative. Abnormal T4 : T8 ratios, in the absence of HTLV III infection, are present in these carriers, in contrast to the heterosexual patients of Mediterranean origin, who have normal T4 : T8 ratios (Novick et al., subm.).

3 Interferon Alpha

Merigan and his colleagues in Stanford California were the first to show that leucocyte interferon was capable of inhibiting hepatitis B virus replication (Greenberg et al. 1976). Limited amounts of interferon were available at this stage and controlled trials could not be undertaken. A randomised controlled trial using leucocyte interferon (Schalm and Heijtink 1982) suffered from the same problems – duration of treatment was too short to produce long-term effects. With the availability of lymphoblastoid and recombinant DNA-produced interferon, longer periods of therapy could be entertained and evaluated in randomised controlled trials.

Initially the drug was given daily and following the studies of Lok et al. (1984a), it became apparent that thrice-weekly interferon was equally effective and better tolerated over periods of treatment of 3 months or more.

The first randomised controlled studies were reported comparing a 1-month course of adenine arabinoside, the most effective form of treatment presently available (Weller et al. 1985), with a 3-month course of lymphoblastoid interferon given thrice weekly at a dosage of $10\,Mu/m^2$ (Lok et al. 1986). Lymphoblastoid interferon gave slightly higher HBe/anti-HBe seroconversion rates, but once again these did not exceed 50% of those patients treated. A further randomised controlled trial compared the effectiveness of 3 and 6 month's therapy – longer term appeared to have no additional beneficial effects (Scully et al., in prep.).

3.1 Factors Influencing Response to Interferon

Once again the data from the Royal Free Hospital controlled trials (Lok et al. 1986) have been analysed in order to determine factors which influence response (Table 2) (Yokosuka et al. 1985). The most important observation is that, in contrast to adenine arabinoside, when interferon is used there are no significant differences in response rates between heterosexual and homosexual carriers. This probably reflects the immunostimulatory effects of interferon, which presumably go some way to correcting the immunodeficiency that occurs in the homosexual group (Novick et al. 1986; Reginstein et al. 1983).

Additional differences in response rate relating to racial and geographic origin, unrelated to sexual preference, are apparent (Thomas and Scully 1985). Patients from Europe show 60–70% response rate to interferon, whereas those from the Far East, predominantly Malaysian, Chinese and Hong Kong Chinese, show virtually no response (Thomas and Scully 1985). Several factors may contribute. It is possible that genetic factors influence the immune response to the virus but, at the present time, this hypothesis is not amenable to further testing. An alternative explanation would be that the mechanism of HBV carriage is different in those infected in these different areas of the world. It is well established that in Northern Europe, the majority of patients are infected in adult life as a result of sexual activities or drug abuse. In contrast the Chinese and Japanese are infected at the time of birth. Preliminary data indicate that the Europeans who becomes HBV carriers have a relative inability to produce alpha interferon and (Ikeda et al. 1986; Abb et al. 1985) it is suggested that this may reduce the effi-

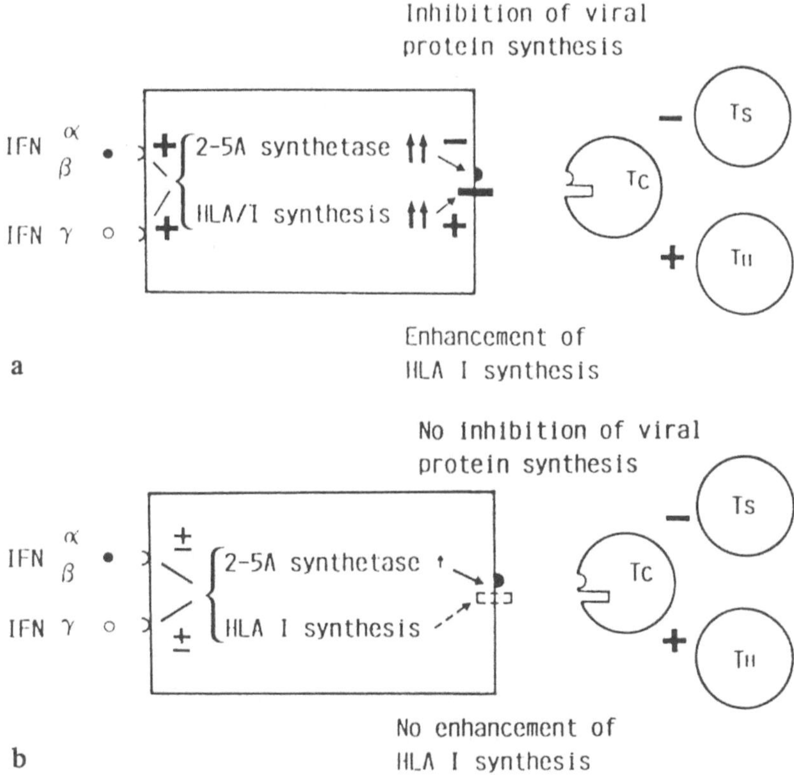

Fig. 2. a Effect of interferon virus-infected cells. α, β and γ-IFN acting through a common receptor activate several enzyme systems, including a 2-5A synthetase. This catalyses production of oligo-adenylates which activate an endogenous ribonuclease leading to cleavage of viral RNA. IFN also causes enhanced expression of HLA class I proteins on the hepatocyte surface facilitating recognition of virus-infected cells by the cellular immune mechanism of the host. **b** Postulated defects occurring in childhood and adult-acquired carrier state. Reduced IFN production leads to failure of HLA display and reduced 2-5A synthetase production

ciency of the hosts antiviral response resulting in a chronic carrier state (Thomas et al. 1986) (Fig. 2). In this group, interferon would be a replacement therapy and good results would be anticipated. In contrast, the Chinese and Japanese, infected at birth, have normal interferon production (Kato et al. 1982), and it seems possible that they have acquired a form of immune tolerance to certain viral proteins. In in vitro cytotoxicity assays, emphasis has been placed on the role of the nucleocapsid protein (Eddleston et al. 1982) as target protein for the host immune response during elimination of virus-infected cells and this is consistent with the observation that chimpanzees immunised with recombinant DNA-produced HBc can be infected, but the infected cells are destroyed, presumably by a cell-mediated immune mechanism, before a significant level of replication, sufficient to give viraemia, has occurred (Iwarson et al. 1985). The infusion of monoclonal anti-HBc to simulate the high titres of anti-HBc present in children born to carrier mothers, has resulted in prolonged infection in chimpanzees

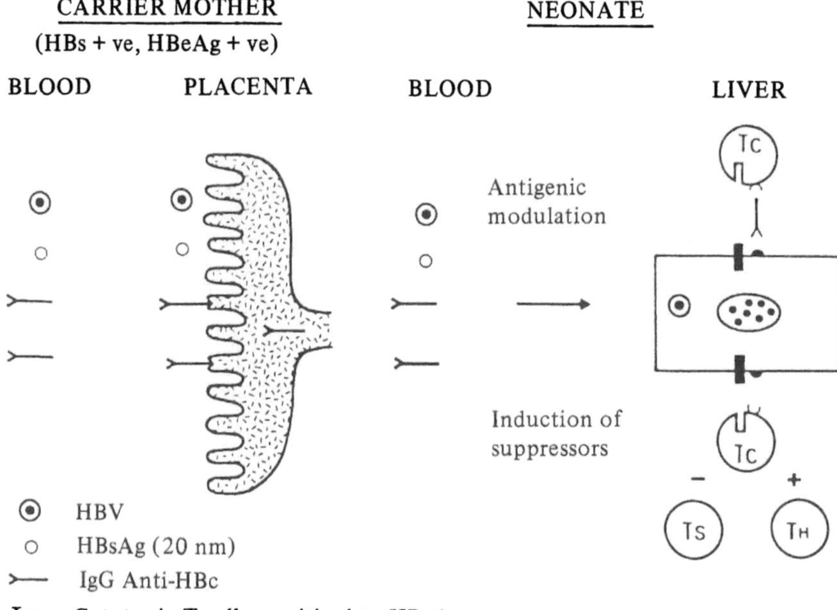

Fig. 3. Postulated mechanisms of the neonatal carrier state. Maternal IgG anti-HBc crosses the placenta into the neonatal circulation. HBV infection of the neonatal liver is thus facilitated as maternal IgG blocks recognition of virus infected cells by cytotoxic T-cells. Early exposure to soluble virus protein may induce a state of antigenic tolerance to the virus with specific suppressor cells inhibiting host defence mechanism.

(Iwarson and Thomas, in prep.). Thus the active transport of anti-HBc across the placenta to the child, along with the immaturity of the immune response at this stage, may result in an inadequate cell-mediated response to the HBc protein, resulting in defective clearance of virus-infected cells (Fig. 3). Interferon has no role in this mechanism, and therefore interferon would be expected to be ineffective.

Another consequence of infection at birth is that when treatment is started in adult life, infection has been present for many years. This is in contrast to the situation present in Western Europe, where patients usually present for treatment within 5 years of the onset of the infection. It is possible that the virus, with time, may influence the ability of the host to mount immune and interferon-related responses. We have recently observed the presence of an interferon-sensitive DNA sequence in the genome of the hepatitis B virus (Thomas et al. 1986). This sequence is also present in the genome of the liver cell (Friedman and Stark 1985) and is involved in the induction, by interferon, of proteins responsible for producing an anti-viral state in the cell. The presence of the homologous sequence in the virus will allow the hepatitis B virus to integrate into these sites in the cell genome, and may render the cell totally or partially unresponsive to interferon. One such interferon-regulated gene is that encoding for the HLA-I protein. The interferon consensus sequence is present up-stream from this gene, and when a cell is exposed to interferon, this sequence may allow an increased rate of transcription of the HLA gene and an increased display of this signal protein on the hepatocyte membrane. This protein, along with the viral protein, acts as a recognition signal to T-cells, allowing them to "kill" the infected hepatocyte. HLA class I proteins are normally present in low density on the liver cell membrane (Thomas et al. 1982), but are increased during an acute hepatitis because of interferon exposure (Pignatelli et al. 1986). We have recently observed that patients undergoing interferon treatment and responding with long-term inhibition of viral replication show a greater increase in serum beta-2 microglobulin than non-responders (Pignatelli et al. 1986). This relative inability to respond to interferon by an increase in HLA synthesis, in patients who ultimately show no long-term benefit from interferon, may stem from integration of HBV sequence into the interferon regulatory sequence within the hosts genome. Thus as the infection continues, the ability of the virus to integrate into the host genome at these sites would progressively render increasing numbers of cells non-responsive to interferon and diminish the chance of successful therapy. This may be what has occurred in patients who have had the infection for a long period of time.

4 Summary

We have reviewed the results of treating over 100 HBV carriers with adenine arabinoside, adenine arabinoside monophosphate and lymphoblastoid interferon.

In the homosexual group of carriers, adenine arabinoside and its monophosphate have no value. However, in this group, lymphoblastoid interferon will produce a response on over 50% of cases. The lack of effectiveness of adenine arabinoside monophosphate in this group may stem from its immunosuppressant properties.

In heterosexual carriers both adenine arabinoside monophosphate and lymphoblastoid interferons are effective in approximately 50–60% of cases. However, the response rate is different in the various racial groups. Northern European and Mediterranean people appear to respond, whereas those from the Far East do not. This may reflect the fact that there are at least two mechanisms by which the chronic carrier state may arise.

In 5–10% of adults, a relative deficiency of alpha interferon production exists (Levin and Hahn 1985) and this defect is found in the majority of HBV carriers in Western Europe. In these, interferon acts as a replacement therapy and excellent results may be obtained if the patient is treated early in the course of the disease. It would appear that as the duration of the infection increases, the virus may integrate into interferon-reactive consensus sites and prevent the cell from responding to interferon.

In patients infected at birth, transplacental anti-HBc appears to modulate the immune response and along with immaturity of the immune system at this age, results in failure to lyse infected cells. These patients do not benefit from interferon treatment: some form of immune manipulation is required.

As in patients with infection acquired in adult life, the presence in the hepatitis B virus genome of an interferon-sensitive site, homologous to that found in the hepatocyte genome, will influence the biological response to interferon.

It is now evident that there are several mechanisms underlying the chronic carrier state, and that in different patients at varying stages of the infection alternative approaches to therapy may be required.

References

Abb J, Zachoval R, Einsenburg J, Pape GR, Zachoral V, Deinhardt F (1985) Production of alpha interferon and interferon gamma by peripheral blood leukocytes from patients with chronic hepatitis B virus infection. J Med Virol 16: 171–176

Bassendine MF, Chadwick RG, Salmeron J, Shipton U, Thomas HC, Sherlok S (1981) Adenine arabinoside therapy in HBsAg-positive chronic liver disease: a controlled study. Gastroenterology 80: 1016–1022

Eddleston AWLF, Mondelli M, Mieli-Vergani G, Williams R (1982) Lymphocyte cytotoxicity to autologous hepatocytes in chronic hepatitis B virus infection. Hepatology 2: 1225–1275

Friedman RL, Stark GR (1985) Interferon induced transcription of HLA and metallothione in genes containing homologous upstream sequence. Nature 314: 637–639

Greenberg HB, Pollard RB, Lutwick LI, Gregory PB, Robinson WS, Merigan TC (1976) Effect of human leukocyte interferon on hepatitis B virus infection in patients with chronic active hepatitis. N Engl J Med 295: 517–522

Hoofnagle JH, Hanson RG, Minuk GY, Pappas SC, Schafer DF, Dusheiko GM, Straus SE, Popper H, Jones AE (1984) Randomised controlled trial of adenine arabinoside monophosphate for chronic type B hepatitis. Gastroenterology 86: 150–157

Ikeda T, Lever AML, Thomas HC (1986) Evidence for a deficiency of IFN production in patients with chronic HBV infection acquired in adult life. Hepatology (in press)

Iwarson S, Tabor E, Thomas HC, Snoy P, Gerety RJ (1985) Protection against hepatitis B virus infection by immunisation with hepatitis B core antigen. Gastroenterology 88: 763–767

Iwarson S, Thomas HC. Passive immunisation with anti-HBc in hepatitis B. (in preparation)

Kato Y, Nakagawa H, Kobayashi K, Hattori N, Hatano K (1982) Interferon production by peripheral lymphocytes in HBsAg-positive liver disease. Hepatology 2: 789–790

Levin S, Hahn T (1985) Interferon deficiency syndrome. Clin Exp Immunol 60: 267–273

Liaw Y, Chu C, Su I, Huang M, Lin D, Chang. Chien C (1983) Clinical and histological events preceeding hepatitis B 'e' antigen seroconversion in chronic type B hepatitis. Gastroenterology 84: 216–219

Lok ASF, Wilson LA, Thomas HC (1984a) Neurotoxicity associated with adenine arabinoside monophosphate in the treatment of chronic hepatitis B virus infection. J Antimicrob Chemother 14: 93–99

Lok ASF, Weller IVD, Karayannis P, Brown D, Fowler MJF, Monjardino J, Thomas HC, Sherlok S (1984b) Thrice weekly lymphoblastoid interferon is effective in inhibiting hepatitis B virus replication. Liver 4: 45–49

Lok ASF, Novick DM, Karayiannis P (1986) A randomised study of the effects of adenine arabinoside 5'-monophosphate (short or long courses) and lymphoblastoid interferon on hepatitis B virus replication. Hepatology (in press)

Novick DM, Lok ASF, Thomas HC (1984) Diminshed responsiveness of homosexual men to antiviral therapy for HBsAg positive chronic liver disease. J Hepatology 1: 29–35

Novick DM, Brown DJ, Lok ASF, Lloyd JC, Thomas HC (1986) Influence of sexual preference and chronic hepatitis B virus infection on T lymphocyte subsets, natural killer activity and suppressor cell activity. J Hepatol (in press)

Perillo RP, Regenstein FG, Bodicky CJ, Campbell CR, Sanders GE, Sunwoo YC (1985) Comparative efficacy of adenine arabinoside 5'-monophosphate and prednisone withdrawal followed by adenine arabinoside 5'-monophosphate in the treatment of chronic active hepatitis type B. Gastroenterology 88: 780–786

Pignatelli M, Waters J, Thomas HC (1986a) Evidence that cytotoxic T-cells sensitised to HBe are responsible for hepatocyte lysis in chronic hepatitis B virus infection. J Hepatology (in press)

Pignatelli M, Waters J, Lever AML, Brown D, Iwarson S, Schaff Z, Gerety R, Thomas HC (1986b) HLA class I antigen on hepatocyte membrane: Increased expression during acute hepatitis B and during interferon therapy of chronic hepatitis B. Hepatology (in press)

Pollard RB, Smith JL, Neal A, Gregory PB, Merigan TC, Robinson WS (1978) The effect of vidarabine on chronic hepatitis B infection. J Am Med Assoc 239: 1648–1650

Realdi G, Alberti A, Rugge M, Bortolotti F, Rigoli AM, Tremolada F, Ruol A (1980) Seroconversion from hepatitis B 'e' antigen to anti-HBe in chronic hepatitis B virus infection. Gastroenterology 79: 195–199

Reginstein FG, Roodman ST, Perillo RP (1983) Immunoregulatory T-cell subsets in chronic hepatitis B virus infection: The influence of homosexuality. Hepatology 31: 951–954

Sacks SL. Scullard GH, Pollard RB, Gregory PB, Robinson WS, Merigan TC (1982). Antiviral treatment of chronic hepatitis B virus infection: pharmokinetics and side effect of interferon and adenine arabinoside alone and in combination. Antimicrob Agents Chemother 21: 91–100

Schalm SW, Heijtink RA (1982) Spontaneous disappearance of viral replication and liver cell inflammation in HBsAg positive chronic active hepatitis: results of a placebo vs interferon trial. Hepatology 2: 791–794

Scullard GH, Pollard RB, Smith JL, Sacks SL. Gregory PB, Robinson WS, Merigan TC (1981) Antiviral treatment of chronic hepatitis B virus infection. 1. Changes in viral markers with interferon combined with adenine arabinoside. J Infect Dis 143: 772–783

Scully LJ, Shein R, Karayiannis P, Thomas HC. Lymphoblastoid interferon therapy of chronic hepatitis B virus infection: a randomised trial of 12 weeks vs 24 weeks of treatment (in preparation)

Smith CI, Weissberg J, Bernhardt L, Gregory PB, Robinson WS, Merigan TC (1983) Acute Dane particle suppression with recombinant leukocyte A interferon in chronic hepatitis B virus infection. J Infect Dis 148: 907–913

Thomas HC, Shipton U, Montano L (1982) The HLA system: its relevance to the pathogenesis of liver disease. In: Popper H, Schaffner F (eds) Progress in liver disease, vol VI. Grune & Stratton, New York, pp 517–527

Thomas HC, Scully LJ (1985) Antiviral therapy in chronic hepatitis B virus infection. Br Med Bull (in press)

Thomas HC, Lever AML, Scully LJ, Pignatelli M (1986) Approaches to the treatment of HBV and delta related liver disease. Semin Liver Dis 6: 34–41

Thomas HC, Pignatelli M, Lever AML (1986) Homology between HBV-DNA and a sequence of regulating the interferon antiviral system: a possible mechanism of persistent infection. J Med Virol 19: 63–69

Trepo C, Hantz O, Ouzan D, Chossegros P, Chevalier P, Berthillon P, Brette R (1984) Therapeutic efficacy of ARA-AMP in symptomatic HBeAg-positive CAH: a randomised placebo control study. Hepatology 4: 1055

Viola LA, Barrison IG, Coleman JC, Paradinas FJ, Fluker JL, Murray-Lyon IM (1981) Natural history of liver disease in chronic hepatitis B surface antigen carriers: a survey of 100 patients from Great Britain. Lancet 2: 1156–1159

Yokosuka O, Omata M, Imazeki F, Hirota K, Mori J, Uchiumi K, Ito Y, Okuda K (1985) Combination of short term prednisolone and adenine arabinoside in the treatment of chronic hepatitis B. A controlled study. Gastroenterology 89: 246–251

Weller IVD, Bassendine MF, Craxi A, Fowler MJF, Monjardino J, Thomas HC, Sherlock S (1982) Successful treatment of HBs and HBeAg-positive chronic liver disease: prolonged inhibition of viral replication by highly soluble adenine arabinoside 5'-monophosphate (ARA-AMP). Gut 23: 717–723

Weller IVD, Carreno V, Fowler MJF, Monjardino J, Makinen D, Varghese Z, Sweny P, Thomas HC, Sherlock S (1983) Acyclovir in hepatitis B antigen-positive chronic liver disease: inhibition of viral replication and transient renal impairment with IV bolus administration. J Antimicrob Chemother 11: 223–231

Weller IVD, Lok ASF, Mindel A, Karayiannis P, Sarah Galphin, Monjardino J, Sherlock S, Thomas HC (1985) A randomised controlled trial of adenine arabinoside 5'-monophosphate (ARA-AMP) in chronic hepatitis B virus infection. Gut 26: 745–751

The Treatment of Chronic Hepatitis Due to Hepatitis B Virus

S. SHERLOCK[1]

1 Introduction

The treatment of chronic active hepatitis due to virus B (HBV) is not as satisfactory as with other forms of chronic hepatitis. The best results follow recognition of the natural history of the disease and whether the problem is that of the infectious, virus-replicating patient or the relatively non-infectious one without viral replication (Sherlock 1985) (Fig. 1). The problem of the individual must be considered, whether it is largely infectivity, symptoms or liver failure. The mode of action of any therapeutic agent must also be understood.

Needle liver biopsy is essential before any therapeutic plan is formulated. A distinction has to be made between chronic persistent hepatitis and chronic active hepatitis. The latter is sub-divided into a mild form which is usually associated with virus B infection, and a more severe type with marked porto-central birdging and rosette formation, which is often associated with the auto-immune type, but can be associated with hepatitis B. A lobular variety is also recognised. Cirrhosis may be found combined with the picture of chronic active hepatitis. In virus B infection, the interpretation of mod-

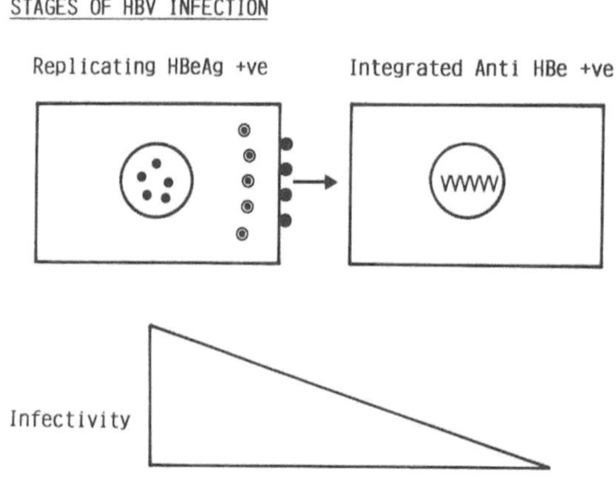

Fig. 1. The natural history of chronic hepatitis B infection. As the patient become, less infectious (conversion of HBeAg-positive to anti-HBe-positive), the viral DNA integrates with that of the host

1   Royal Free Hospital Hampstead N.W.3, School of Medicine University of London, London, United Kingdom

Viral Hepatitis, ed. by F. Callea et al.
© Springer-Verlag Berlin Heidelberg 1986

est piecemeal necrosis and erosion of the limiting plate of hepatocytes can be overemphasised. The presence of severe chronic active hepatitis with cirrhosis will obviously make treatment more urgent.

2 Markers of Infectivity

It is essential to test not only for hepatitis B surface antigen (HBsAg), but also for the serum markers of viral replication which are constituents of the core of hepatitis B virus. The most usual core antigen is HBeAg, which with its antibody, anti-HBe, can be tested by commercial kits. Advances in molecular biology now allow measurement of serum hepatitis B polymerase (HBV-DNAp) and also serum HBV-DNA by molecular hybridisation with ^{32}P-labelled cloned HBV-DNA (Weller et al. 1982a; Sherlock and Thomas 1983). Such sophisticated techniques, however, are not yet generally available. During chronic HBV infection, there is a phase of high-level viral replication, when the patient is HBeAg- and HBV-DNA-positive. This is followed by a phase of chronic HBs antigenemia without evidence of viral replication, when there is anti-HBe in the serum. During the period of HBe antigenemia, the patient is highly infectious, and there is more rapid progression of hepatic inflammatory activity. Spontaneous clearance of HBeAg occurs relatively infrequently, and antiviral agents are used to accelerate the process. The conversion of the infectious to non-infectious stage increases with age. The patient is more likely to be serum anti-HBe-positive, and HBV-DNA-negative when the hepatic histological picture has progressed from chronic hepatitis to cirrhosis (Craxi et al. 1983). The management of a patient who is HBeAg- and HBV-DNA-positive will clearly differ from the patient who is anti-HBe-positive and lacks serum HBV-DNA.

At some stage the hepatitis B viral genome integrates with that of the host, so that the host DNA is coding for viral DNA (Bréchot et al. 1981; Shafritz et al. 1981). When this has happened, antiviral therapy will be unavailing. Integration is a precursor of primary liver cancer.

3 General Measures

The patient must be counselled concerning personal infectivity. This is particularly important if he is HBeAg-positive. Counselling is particularly important in relation to sexual contacts, blood donations or accidental lacerations which may occur during his occupation, for instance, surgeon, dentist or worker in oncology or renal unit. Close family and sexual contacts should be checked for HBcAb, and if negative, hepatitis B vaccination should be offered.

The patient should be encouraged to lead a normal life without becoming excessively fatigued. Bed rest is not helpful. Physical fitness in encouraged by graduated exercises. Alcohol excess should be avoided, as this enhances the effects of HBsAg carriage (Villa et al. 1982). However, one or two glasses of wine or beer a day are allowed if this is part of the patient's lifestyle and if it is believed that he does not abuse alcohol.

Diet should be normal unless the patient has ascites, when sodium should be restricted, or hepatic encephalopathy, when dietary protein intake should be reduced.

The value of vitamin supplements or hepato-protectives has not been confirmed by controlled trials. The majority of patients with chronic hepatitis B lead normal lives. Strong reassurance from the physician will prevent introspection by the patient.

4 Aims of Therapy

The aims are to eradicate the hepatitis B virus, to lower infectivity and to improve chronic liver disease. The eradication of hepatitis B as shown by the development of a negative HBsAg test is extremely rare with any form of therapy. Even after cessation of detectable HBV replication, HBsAg is produced. This suggests that viral DNA has integrated into the host cell genome even at a relatively early stage of chronic infection. Lowering of infectivity achieved spontaneously or by antiviral agents is shown by disappearance of serum HBeAg and of HBV-DNA.

Improvement of liver function may be achieved following antiviral therapy. A spontaneous remission in clinical .and biochemical evidence of active disease is usually heralded or accompanied by the disappearance of HBeAg and HBV-DNA from the serum. The stage of viral integration with the host is uncertain, but the chance of detecting integrated HBV-DNA sequences in the hepatocyte is much higher in long-standing infections. Treatment early, before stable clones of integrated HBV-DNA are established, might lead to complete eradication of the virus. Early antiviral treatment would also be beneficial in reducing the activity of chronic hepatitis, and so the development of cirrhosis. Despite viral integration with the host, the absence of cirrhosis would make the development of primary liver cancer less likely.

5 Antiviral Therapy for the HBeAg-Positive Patient

Pre-testing for serum HBeAg and anti-HBe is essential. Antiviral treatment must be considered for the HBeAg-positive, particularly if likely to be a serious source of infection to contacts. Antivirals under consideration include adenine arabinoside, the interferons and acyclovir.

Adenine Arabinoside (ARA-A) is a synthetic purine nucleoside with a broad spectrum of antiviral activity against DNA viruses. In HBeAg-positive patients, ARA-A alone can produce permanent inhibition of HBV-DNAp activity with loss of HBeAg and decrease in HBsAg concentrations and aspartate transaminases. ARA-A has a low toxicity, but its use is limited by insolubility and the need for continuous intravenous administration. Adenine arabinoside 5-monophosphate (ARA MP) is at least 400 times more water-soluble. It is suitable for intramuscular or intravenous administration. Intramuscular ARA-AMP, given short-term (9–14 days), produced only transient inhibition of viral replication (Weller et al. 1982c). In those treated with a smaller dose for longer (3–5 weeks) serum HBV-DNA polymerase and HBV-DNA activity and HBeAg were lost, anti-HBe developed and HBsAg concentrations decreased (Weller et al. 1985). In a study of 15 patients given ARA-AMP, all showed inhibition of HBV-DNAp. Only 6, however, showed long-term disappearance of HBV-DNA and HBV-DNAp (Gregory

1984). Disappearance of HBeAg and appearance of anti-HBe was delayed for 180 days; HBsAg persisted, although transient reductions of serum HBV-DNA are usual, conversion of HBeAg to HBeAb is not common (Gregory 1984). The most recent results from the Royal Free Hospital, London, showed that only 10 of 46 (22%) patients lost HBeAg in 1 year (Scully et al. 1985). Another recent, small, controlled study also showed disappointing results (Hoofnagle 1984). A transient rise in serum aspartate transaminase after treatment in those who seroconverted may indicate that hepatocyte lysis is involved in the process. The serum aspartate transaminase values later fell. Twice-daily intramuscular ARA-AMP in a dose of 5 mg per kilogram per day for 8 weeks may be an appropriate course.

High doses of ARA-AMP are associated with thrombocytopenia. Renal function is preserved. Fever and malaise are common. The most serious side-effect is a muscular pain syndrome with stiffening of the muscles affecting predominantly the lower limbs, which complicates long-term therapy (Gregory 1984).

Interferons could be useful against HBV infections in various ways. Firstly, they are antiviral at multiple sites. Secondly, they are anticellular and anti-tumor agents affecting cell division, protein synthesis and DNA synthesis. Finally, they affect the immune system, increasing T-cell cytotoxicity, macrophages and natural killer cells. Interferons act primarily on virion production and not on the manufacture of incomplete HBsAg particles (Robinson and Garcia 1985). They enhance HLA antigen hepatocyte display.

Interferon deficiency may predispose to the development of the chronic carrier state arising after hepatitis B viral infection in adulthood. In chronic hepatitis B viral infection there may be failure of recognition of HLA markers displayed on the hepatocyte membrane to which the immune response is directed; interferons may enhance such display (Ikeda et al. 1985). In addition, interleukin-2 (IL-2) activity is decreased in patients with HBV-related chronic liver disease. Interferons may increase interleukin-2 receptor expression on peripheral blood mononuclear cell (Nouri-Aria et al. 1985).

The interferons used successfully to treat chronic hepatitis B viral infections are leucocyte, lymphoblastoid and more recently, α-1 interferon prepared from *E. coli* using recombinant DNA technology. Some patients will respond to interferon treatment, but others do not. This may be related to duration of infection and how far integration of host and viral DNA has taken place in the hepatocyte nucleus.

Human leucocyte interferon alone or in combination with ARA-A, has, in some patients with chronic hepatitis, produced permanent inhibition of viral replication. This is shown by loss of HBV-DNA and seroconversion from HBeAg to anti-HBe. Lymphoblastoid interferon (Wellferon from Wellcome laboratories) is a mixture of α-interferons produced by stimulation of human lymphoblastoid cell line with Sendai virus. It inhibits HBV replication when given by daily intramuscular injection or by continuous intravenous infusion(Weller et al. 1982a). It is possible to give a smaller dose less often. Intramuscular interferon given three times a week in a relatively small dose resulted in suppression of viral replication (Lok et al. 1984, 1986). This was associated with a marked reduction in the "flu-like" side effects associated with daily administration of larger doses of interferon. The rise in transaminase values during treatment may have reflected lysis of infected hepatocytes. Transaminase values fell in those who showed persistent inhibition of viral replication (Fig. 2).

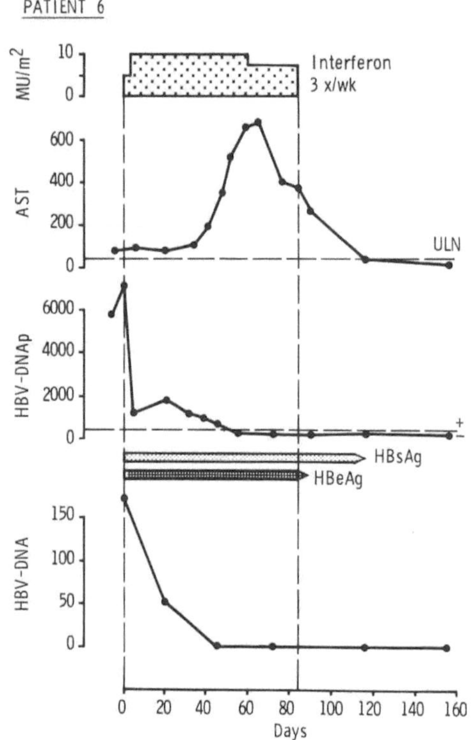

Fig. 2. Thrice-weekly interferon for 84 days resulted in a rise in aspartate transaminase, a fall in HBV-DNA and HBV-DNA polymerase with a loss of HBeAg and HBsAg. (Lok et al. 1984)

Recombinant leucocyte A interferon can be used, the maximum antiviral effect being below the maximum tolerated dose (Omata et al. 1985). In a small controlled trial of recombinant interferon, 6 of 14 carriers showed sustained loss of HBeAg and HBV-DNA and 4 subsequently lost HBsAg (Dusheiko et al. 1985).

The present results from the Royal Free Hospital, using lymphoblastoid interferon, show that 19 of 31 (61%) treated patients lost HBeAg in 1 year. Results from Madrid have shown a 58% loss of HBe antigen (Porres et al. 1985).

The use of antivirals, especially interferon in hepatitis B carriers will depend on the availability of agents in large quantities and at low cost. Recombinant techniques of preparation must be extended. The patients must be compliant, as at least 4—8 weeks of intramuscular therapy are usually needed. About two thirds will achieve permanent suppression of viral replication. More studies of the effect on the natural history of the disease are necessary using a treated and control group and with more clearly defined patient groups.

Acyclovir (Acycloguanosine) inhibits Herpes simplex virus in vitro and in vivo, its action being dependent on phosphorylation by a virus-coded thymidine kinase. Two patients with chronic hepatitis B liver disease were treated with 10 and 15 mg per kilogram acyclovir intravenously 8-hourly for 5—7 days (Weller et al. 1982d). They showed inhibition of DNAp and HNV-DNA. More work is needed using this agent for longer periods. It has the disadvantage of intravenous administration.

6 Corticosteroids Followed by Antiviral Therapy

Corticosteroid therapy in the HBeAg-positive patient enhances viral replication. Its withdrawal induces immune stimulation with temporary loss of hepatitis B viral markers such as DNA polymerase and hepatitis B e antigen (Scullard et al. 1979; Weller et al. 1982d). Antiviral therapy given during the immune stimulation period following prednisone withdrawal might be more effective than when given alone. In one such trial, prednisone 40 mg, tapering over 8 weeks, was followed by adenine arabinoside monophosphate for 28 days. This resulted in 72% response in hepatitis e antigen clearance rate (Perrillo et al. 1985). In another study, 6 of 9 (57%) of e antigen-positive patients receiving combination therapy lost e antigen, compared with only 4 of 24 (17%) receiving either adenine arabinoside monophosphate alone or prednisolone alone (Yokosuka et al. 1985). Such therapy has to be given cautiously, too abrupt cessation of prednisolone may be followed by such marked immune stimulation that acute hepatocellular necrosis ensues.

7 Factors Affecting Trials of Antiviral Therapy

At the present time, results of trials are extremely difficult to interpret (Gregory 1984). The numbers in any one trial are very small and many lack controls. The regimes differ, both in duration and dose, and the type of antiviral agent varies. This particularly applies to the interferons; the relative efficacy of lymphoblastoid versus recombinant remains uncertain.

In addition, the patients being treated vary. Perhaps the most important factor is the time when the infection was acquired. Those infected in early childhood are likely to be well on the way to viral DNA integration with host DNA before antiviral treatment is given and so do not respond. This may explain why the Oriental and Southern European peoples, who have a high infection rate in early life, do poorly with antiviral therapy. Caucasians, developing the disease later and being treated earlier, achieve better results. If the patient has a deficiency in cell-mediated immunity, results will be poor. Hence, homosexuals respond rarely to therapy and especially to ARA-AMP. This is particularly so if they are homosexuals who have AIDS antibody (anti-HTLV III). In London, 40% of homosexuals carrying HBsAg are also HTLV III-positive. This group is all HBeAg-positive with high serum HBV-DNA levels. The underlying chronic hepatitis is mild, serum transaminases are low. They do not respond to antiviral therapy (Caruso et al. 1985).

8 The Anti-HBe Positive Patient

Patients who fall into this group tend to be older and have more advanced liver disease. If they are asymptomatic or with only mild symptoms, conservative measures are all that should be offered. Advanced age, concomitant disease such as diabetes or a history of many years of non-progressive liver disease also contraindicate treatment. Such patients should have 6-monthly clinical and biochemical checks with biopsies as indicated to assess progress.

Prednisolone therapy must be considered for those who are symptomatic, e antigen-negative and where liver biopsy shows chronic active hepatitis, with or without cirrhosis. In the e antigen-positive patient, corticosteroids will increase viral replication (Robinson and Garcia 1985; Weller et al. 1982d) and may have a deleterious effect (Wu et al. 1982). There is some evidence in the anti-HBe patient that perpetuation of the chronic hepatitis may be immunologically mediated. Prednisolone therapy is started in a dose of 30 mg for 1 week and reduced to a maintenance of 10–15 mg daily which is continued for 3 months. Life may be prolonged (Sagnelli et al. 1983). If there is no clinical or biochemical evidence of benefit, the drug is stopped. If improvement ensues, it may be continued, usually for a period of some 2 years. It cannot be discounted that prednisolone may increase the chances of later hepatocellular carcinoma. Such therapy must in no sense be regarded as desirable. Indeed, it is indicated only if the disease is rapidly progressive and/or other available therapy has failed (Conn et al. 1982).

9 Treatment of Delta (HDV) Infection

Delta superinfection accelerates the progress of chronic hepatitis B (Smedile et al. 1982). There have been only limited attempts to control delta infection using antiviral therapy. Five patients with chronic delta infection were treated with lymphoblastoid interferon (10 mega units/m^2, thrice-weekly for 3 months) and followed for 1 year (Farci et al. 1985). Three lost delta RNA from their serum, and two showed a marked fall. These changes persisted for 1 year, but in one patient, HDV-RNA returned and a liver biopsy showed delta viral antigen. Serum transaminase values improved in only three. Clearly, these observations must be extended. Relapses after therapy seem likely.

References

Bréchot C, Hadchouel M, Scotto J. Fonck M, Potet F, Vyas GN, Tiollais P (1981) State of hepatitis B virus DNA in hepatocytes of patients with hepatitis B surface antigen-positive and negative liver disease. Proc Natl Acad Sci USA 78: 3906

Caruso L, Weber JN, Forster GE, Scully L, Harris TRW, Thomas HC (1985) Effects of HTLV III virus infection on replication, severity of liver disease and response to interferon in chronic hepatitis B virus carriers. J Hepatol Suppl 2: 207

Craxi A, Weller IVD, Bassendine MF, Fowler MJ, Monjardino J, Thomas HC, Sherlock S (1983) Relationship between HBV-specific DNA polymerase in chronic HBV infection: factors determining selection of patients and outcome of antiviral therapy. Gut 24: 143

Conn HO, Maddrey WC, Soloway RD (1982) The detrimental effects or adrenocorticosteroid therapy in HBsAg-positive chronic hepatitis: facts or artefact? Hepatology 2: 885

Dusheiko G, Dibisceglie A, Bowyer S, Sachs E, Ridche EM, Schoub B, Kew M (1985) Recombinant leukocyte interferon treatment of chronic hepatitis B. Hepatology 5: 556

Farci P, Karayiannis P, Smedile A, Gerin J, Thomas HC (1985) Chronic delta virus infection: response to lymphoblastoid interferon. J Hepatol 1, Suppl 2: 227

Gregory PB (1984) Antivirals in chronic hepatitis B − problems of small clinical trials. Gastroenterology 86: 201

Hoofnagle JH, Hanson RG, Minuk GY, Pappas Sc, Shafer DF, Dusheiko GM, Straus SE, Popper H, Jones EA (1984) Randomized controlled trial of adenine arabinoside 5-monophosphate for chronic type B hepatitis. Gastroenterology 86: 150

Ikeda T, Lever AML, Thomas HC (1985) Deficient production of interferon alpha predispose to chronic hepatitis B infection. J Hepatol Suppl 2: 256

Lok ASF, Karayiannis P, Brown D, Fowler MJ, Monjardino J, Thomas HC, Sherlock S (1984) Thrice weekly lymphoblastoid interferon is effective in inhibiting hepatitis B virus replication. Liver 4: 45

Lok ASF, Novick DM Karayiannis P (1986) A randomized study of the effects of adenine arabinoside 5-monophosphate (short or long courses) and lymphoblastoid interferon on hepatitis B virus replication. Hepatology (in press)

Nouri-Aria KT, Magrin S, Anderson GJM, Alexander GJM, Eddlestone ALWF, Williams R (1985) Interleukin-2 receptor expression before and after in vitro and interferon treatment in chronic hepatitis B virus (HBV) infection. J Hepatol Suppl 2: 298

Omata M, Imazeki F, Yokosuka O, Ito Y, Uchiumi K, Mori T, Okuda K (1985) Recombinant leukocyte A interferon treatment in patients with chronic hepatitis B virus infection. Gastroenterology 88: 870

Perrillo RP, Regenstein FG, Bodicky CJ, Campbell CR, Sanders GE, Sunwoo YC (1985) Comparative efficiency of adenine arabinoside 5'-monophosphate and prednison withdrawal followed by adenine arabinoside 5'-monophosphate in the treatment of chronic active hepatitis type B. Gastroenterology 88: 780

Porres JC, Carreno V, Mora I, Gutiez G, Quiroga JA, Bartolomè J, Cortez J, Hernandez J (1985) Changes of viral markers and liver histology in patients treated during six months with recombinant interferon. J Hepatol Suppl 2: 312

Robinson WS, Garcia G (1985) Interferon and hepatitis B. Hepatology 5: 336

Sagnelli E, Piccino F, Manzillo G, Felaco FM, Filippini P, Maio G, Pasquale G, Izzo CM (1983) Effect of immunosuppressive therapy on HBsAg-positive active hepatitis in relation to presence or absence of HBeAg and anti-HBe. Hepatology 3: 690

Scullard GH, Robinson WS, Merigan TC, Robinson WS, Gregory PB (1979) The effect of immunosuppressive therapy on hepatitis B viral infection in patients with chronic hepatitis. Gastroenterology 77: 43A

Scully LJ, Shein R, Lok ASF, Thomas HC (1985) Factors determining response rate to antiviral therapy in chronic hepatitis B infection. J Hepatol Suppl 2: 328

Sherlock S, Thomas HC (1983) Hepatitis B virus infection: the impact of molecular biology. Hepatology 3: 455

Sherlock S, (1985) Chronic hepatitis. In: Diseases of the liver and biliary system, 7th ed, Blackwell-Mosby, Oxford St. Louis, p 295

Shafritz DA, Shouval D, Sherman HI, Hadziyannis ST, Kew M (1981) Integration of hepatitis B virus DNA into the genome of liver cells in chronic liver disease and hepatocellular carcinoma. New Engl J Med 35: 1067

Smedile A, Farci P, Verme G, Caredda F, Cargnel A, Caporaso N, Dentico P, Trepo C, Opolon P, Gimson A, Vergani D, Williams R, Rizzetto M (1982) Influence of delta infection on severity of hepatitis B. Lancet 2: 945

Villa E, Rubbiani L, Barchi T, Ferret I, Grisendi A, De Palma M, Bellentani S, Manenti F (1982) Susceptibility of chronic symtomless HBsAg carriers to ethanol-induced hepatic damage. Lancet ii: 1243

Weller IVD, Fowler MF, Monjardino J, Thomas HC (1982a) The detection of HBV-DNA in serum by molecular hybridisation−a more sensitive method for the detection of complete HBV particles. J Med Virol 9: 273

Weller IVD, Carreno V, Fowler MF, Monjardino J, Makinen D, Thomas HC, Sherlock S (1982b) Acyclovir inhibits hepatitis B virus replication in man. Lancet i: 273

Weller IVD, Bassendine MF, Craxi A, Fowler MJ, Monjardino J, Thomas HC, Sherlock S (1982c) Successful treatment of HBs and HBeAg positive chronic liver disease: prolonged inhibition of viral replication by highly soluble adenine arabinoside 5-monophosphate (ARA-AMP). Gut 23: 717

Weller IVD, Bassendine MF, Murray A, Craxi A, Thomas HC, Sherlock S, (1982d) The effects of prednisolone/azathioprine in chronic hepatitis B viral infection. Gut 23: 650

Weller IVD, Lok ASF, Mindel A, Karayiannis P, Galpin S, Monjardino J, Sherlock S, Thomas HC (1985) Randomised controlled trial of adenine arabinoside 5-monophosphate (ARA-AMP) in chronid hepatitis-B virus infection. Gut 26: 745

Wu Pc, Lai CL, Lam KC, Ho J (1982) Prednisolone in HBsAg-positive chronic active hepatitis: histologic evaluation in a controlled prospective study. Hepatology 2: 777

Yokosuka O, Omata M, Imazeki F, Hirota K, Mori I, Uchiumi K, Ito Y, Okuda K (1985) Combination of short-term prednisolone and adenine arabinoside in the treatment of chronic hepatitis B. A controlled study. Gastroenterology 89: 246

Hepatitis B Virus and Hepatocellular Carcinoma

R.N.M. MacSWEEN[1]

1 Introduction

While this review will critically examine the evidence that hepatitis B (HBV) is causally related to hepatocellular carcinoma (HCC), we must not forget that other factors may also be involved. In our current state of knowledge, any discussion of hepatocellular carcinogenesis must also consider the role of certain chemicals and toxins, alcohol and hormones, and the significance of cirrhosis. Complex inter-relationships exist between these various factors. Some of these will be referred to as appropriate to the specific topic of hepatitis B oncogenesis. For more extensive accounts, however, reference should be made to the list of publications appended to this paper. These, in the main, are review articles from which, however, the original publications are readily obtained.

The evidence implicating an oncogenic role for HBV comes from several different lines of investigation and these are summarised in Table 1. Each of these is now examined in greater detail.

Table 1. HBV Infection and hepatocellular carcinoma

1. Retrospective epidemiological studies
2. Family studies: perinatal transmission
3. Prospective epidemiological studies
4. HBV antigen expression in tumour and liver
5. Integration of HBV DNA in tumour cell genome
6. Mechanisms of HBV carcinogenesis
7. Animal models

2 Retrospective Epidemiological Studies

On a world-wide basis, the prevalence of chronic carriers of HBV and the incidence of HCC correlate closely, such that a map showing the distribution of the former matches that of the latter almost exactly. There is apparently no country in the world which has a high incidence of HCC and a low prevalence of HBsAg carriers. Even in countries

1 University of Glasgow, Department of Pathology, Western Infirmary, Glasgow G11, 6NT, Scotland

Viral Hepatitis, ed. by F. Callea et al.
© Springer-Verlag Berlin Heidelberg 1986

with a low tumour incidence, a disproportionately high frequency of HBV infection is found among patients with tumour. This variation in tumour incidence in, e.g., Greece and variations within different ethnic groups in the same locality, e.g., Los Angeles have been positively correlated with differences in HBV infection rates. The geographical distribution of HCC favours an environmental aetiological agent. The parallel distribution of chronic HBsAg carrier suggests that HBV could be one such environmental factor. However, the possibility of genetic factors playing a role has also to be considered. No good evidence in favour of this has emerged and studies on MHC antigen status and liver cell carcinoma have not provided any evidence of a close association.

It is of more interest, however, that the universal male to female preponderance of HCC is not entirely explicable on the basis of chronic hepatitis B infection being commoner in males. In South Africa (Kew 1984) the male to female carrier rate is 2 : 1, but the corresponding ratio for HCC is 5 or 6 : 1. Kew and his colleagues, in a comparison of age-matched patients with HCC, found that in females the rates of active or present infection with HBV was the same as in males. It would thus appear that HBV may prove to be equally oncogenic in males and females.

Numerous studies in many countries have conclusively shown a much higher frequency of HBV markers in patients with HCC than in controls. Initially based on seropositivity for HBsAg using relatively insensitive methods, the evidence has become compellingly impressive as more sensitive techniques have been developed, and the different antigen/antibody systems of the virus have been investigated. The HBsAg positivity rate in a great number of studies of tumour patients has ranged from 40–80%, contrasting with rates of < 15% in matched controls. The strong association of HCC with HBs antigenaemia rather than with HBsAb status indicated that the correlation was with active rather than with past infection. This is further confirmed by the finding of HBeAb in approximately 50% of tumour patients, while serum HBV-DNA and DNA polymerase are demonstrable in a small number of patients; in a study of 90 tumour patients, Kew (1984) found that 58 (64%) were seronegative for HBeAg, HBV-DNA and DNA polymerase. This suggests that there is little or no active HBV replication in HCC patients. However, the possibility that the tumour per se suppresses viral replication has to be borne in mind. No particular sub-type of HBV (adw, adr, ayw or ayr) has been associated with tumour, and thus an oncogenic strain apparently does not exist.

3 Family Studies: Perinatal Transmission

Clusters of HBsAg-positive patients with liver cell carcinoma and/or cirrhosis have been reported mainly in the Far East and Japan. Siblings and family members across several generations have been involved, and the pattern of HBsAg positivity has indicated transmission from mother to child. Perinatal transmission from mother to child is now accepted for more than 40% of HBsAg carriers in high-incidence areas.

These family study have suggested the possibility that maternal transmission per se may be related to an increased risk of HCC. Evidence from Senegal and Taiwan suggests that the risk of developing HCC may be increased among carriers infected from their mothers; in these studies the mothers of HCC cases had a much higher frequency of HBsAg positivity than controls. The possibility that HBV infection will lead to a chronic carrier state is inversely related to the age at infection; in newborns the risk is of the order of 80–90%, whereas in adults the corresponding figure is 10%. It seems that this reflects immaturity of the immune system in the youngest age group. However, it does suggest that liver cancer is more likely to develop in those who contract HBV infection at a very early age and thus become carriers.

4 Prospective Epidemiological Studies

These perhaps provide the best evidence of a role for HBV in HCC. The studies by Beasley and his colleagues in Taiwan commenced in 1975 and have involved 22,707 male government employers in whom the follow-up period was 6.2 years/man through December 31st 1983 (Beasley and Hwang 1984). In these studies they showed that the relative risk factor of developing HCC was 217 among the 3454 (15.2%) of HBsAg-positive carriers; 116 tumours developed during this period, of which 113 were in HBsAg-positive patients and 3 among 19,253 non-carriers; all 3 were HBcAb-positive and 2 also had HBsAb. The overall annual incidence of tumour in the study population was 82.5 cases/100,000, but in the carriers the corresponding figure was 527.3.

On the basis of more detailed analysis of their data, Beasley and his colleagues found that:

a) the excessive risk of HCC may be lost when the HBsAg carrier state disappears, i.e. when sero-conversion occurs.
b) there was a fivefold increased tumour risk in HBsAg-positive cases with proven cirrhosis; this is probably an underestimate of the combined risk if one bears in mind the fact that, of patients with tumour, less than 15% do not have cirrhosis and that cirrhosis is frequently asymptomatic until an advanced stage.
c) the life-time risk of death from liver cell carcinoma and/or cirrhosis in carriers approached 50%.
d) a previous history of hepatitis increased the tumour risk three-fold, and the risk was increased by a similar factor in carriers with increased levels of IgM class anti-HBc.

Similar evidence of the increased risk of HCC for HBsAg carriers has come from prospective Japanese and Hawaiian studies, the annual tumour incidence in the former being 396/100,000.

Although the Taiwan studies showed an increased tumour risk when cirrhosis was present, they did not clarify the relationhsip between cirrhosis and tumour. Of 30 HBsAg-negative patients with cirrhosis of unknown aetiology who entered the study, none subsequently developed liver cancer. The data obtained by Beasley's group was not inconsistent with the possibility that the cirrhosis and tumour were both caused by HBV and developed independently. In South Africa, Kew (1984) found that the prevalence of cirrhosis in HCC patients was not related to age, nor were the patients with cirrhosis significantly older than those without cirrhosis. Kew considers that these observations indicate that the tumour is not a direct complication of cirrhosis; the tumour and cirrhosis may be different end-results of the same aetiological agent and malignant transformation takes the same length of time whether or not cirrhosis is present. In HBsAg-positive patients with cirrhosis and tumour, the cirrhosis is usually of a macronodular pattern. In addition, there is usually only minimal chronic active hepatitis, this also reflecting the absence of active viral replication.

There is now no good evidence that cirrhosis per se should be regarded as a pre-malignant lesion with neoplasia supervening hyperplasia. When there is a low HCC tumour incidence and a low prevalence of chronic HBsAg carriers, the tumour/cirrhosis relationship may be different. In these situations cirrhosis would act in a "promoter" role, continued liver-cell necrosis and regeneration increasing cell sensitivity to potential carcinogens (Kew and Popper 1984).

5 HBV Antigen Expression

Whereas HBsAg and, less frequently, HBcAg have been readily demonstrable in the "normal" hepatocytes of tumour-bearing livers, these antigens are infrequently found within tumour cells, and this usually in the better differentiated ones. In several tumour cell lines HBsAg production, however, has been found, the material secreted being essentially similar to the surface antigen found in the serum of infected patients. In studies using serum-free medium and PLC/PRF/5 cells, HBsAg production has been reported and it is currently thought that in this cell line and in others most of the viral genome is present, thus affording valuable models for further investigation of viral integration and expression (Gerber and Thung 1985). In one recent study Suzuki et al. (1985) reported the production of complete viral particles by tumour cells. This will require confirmation, the current general view being that HBV replication becomes defective during malignant transformation.

6 Integration of HBV-DNA into Tumour Cell Genome

HBV-DNA sequences have now been detected in the large majority of liver-cell cancers developing in HBsAg-positive patients. In a number of studies, integrated HBV-DNA has also been demonstrated in tumour cells from patients positive for HBs antibody. Bréchot and his colleagues (Bréchot et al. 1984, 1985), in hitherto unconfirmed reports, have also reported integration in tumours arising in patients who were sero-negative for all HBV markers.

The integration patterns described appear to be unique for each tumour, suggesting monoclonality of the tumour cells. However, the integration into the cell genome appears to be random, with extensive rearrangement, deletions, duplications and inverted duplications (Gerber and Thung 1985). In the viral genome, integration involves either the single-stranded or the overlap region, and the 5' "cohesive end" of the viral genome may then be functionally important in integration. However, there is neither evidence for a specific cellular integration site nor whether specific sites in HBV-DNA regularly form certain sites in cellular DNA.

The integration of viral DNA is regarded as a critical event in viral oncogenesis and the evidence that HBV-DNA integration occurs in HCC is therefore of considerable importance.

7 Mechanisms of HBV Carcinogenesis

While the foregoing account provides compelling evidence for a casual role of HBV in liver-cell carcinoma, the precise mechanism(s) involved in tumour transformation remain(s) uncertain. There is no evidence that HBV infection results in mutation of cellular genes that would result in cell transformation, i.e. "hit and run" mechanism. Similarly, there is no evidence that HBV carries its own oncogene or oncogenes that lead to induction of tumours in vivo or will produce transformation of cells in vitro. Finally, it has not been shown that the cellular sequences flanking viral inserts contain cellular oncogenes or that their expression is altered in HBV-infected cells. Thus a "promotor-insertion" mechanism of HBV carcinogenesis cannot yet be implicated.

8 Animal Models

This topic is discussed elsewhere in this issue. In both the woodchuck and the Pekin duck model, integration of the corresponding Hepadna virus DNA has been shown and the oncogenic role of the virus in these species is now generally accepted. It is worth noting that while chimpanzees are susceptible to HBV infection, viral DNA integration does not occur in them and, to date, no liver-cell tumours have been reported in chronic carriers.

9 Conclusions

The prospective studies from Taiwan and Japan are strong evidence that HBV can directly cause liver-cell cancer. As Beasley and Hwang (1984) point out, establishment of a high relative risk in a prospective epidemiological study is second only to excess risk established in a formal experiment in terms of providing a cause-and-effect relationship. Their data would suggest that HBV may be able to produce HCC alone. The studies on HBV-DNA integration have provided critical evidence, at the molecular level, of possible viral carcinogenesis in liver-cell cancer; the precise mechanisms of oncogenesis are not, however, clear. The possibility that in hepatic oncogenesis non-viral factors are also involved cannot be excluded. Sherman and Shafritz (1984) have suggested that liver-cell carcinogenesis is a multi-stage process (Fig. 1). They hypothesise that HBV-DNA integration occurs, perhaps during the acute infection or at some later stage of the chronic carrier state. Whereas cells in which viral replication occurs are removed by host immune mechanisms, cells in which HBV-DNA is integrated may escape immune surveillance and preferentially persist. Normal cell division, or accelerated cell division due, e.g., to liver-cell injury from toxins, other viruses or whatever, could result, at Stage I, in an increase in the number of cells containing integrated HBV-DNA. Subsequent further selection of a clone or clones of cells containing integrated viral DNA could result in focal growth of such transformed cells (Stage II) with eventual emergence of liver-cell cancer. This multi-stage model of HCC development is one in which, at a number of points, interplay between the virus, host factors and other exogenous factors could occur. These factors and possible interaction between them are the subject of continued intensive investigations.

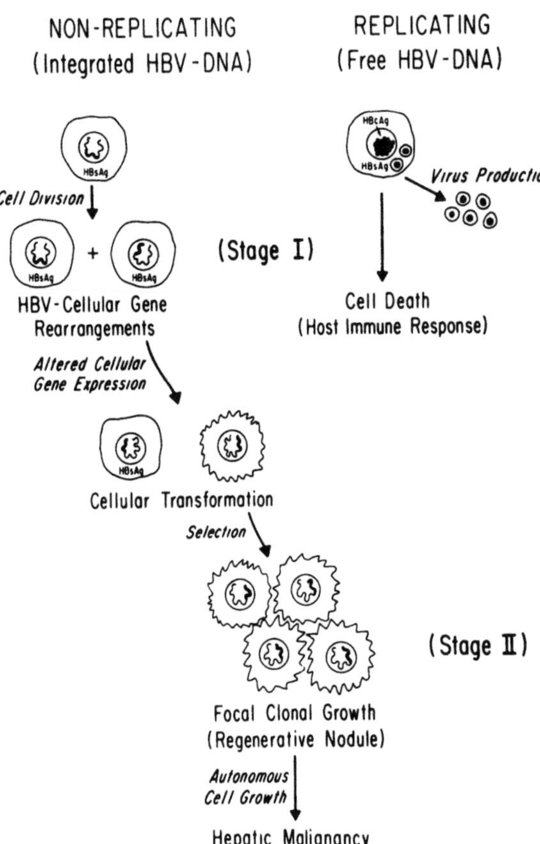

Fig. 1. Diagrammatic representation of a hypothesis encompassing both viral and non-viral factors in the pathogenesis of liver-cell carcinoma. The hypothesis implies a change in the state of integrated HBV-DNA during persistent infection by the virus. (Sherman and Shafritz 1984)

If criteria for viral malignancy are applied to HBV, it is clear from the preceding account that a number are already met either fully or in part. Transformation experiments with HBV-DNA have been unsuccessful, but the animal models have provided evidence that the Hepadna viruses can induce liver-cell tumours. Much is expected of HBV vaccination programmes, not least the possibility of eliminating a large proportion of primary liver-cell cancers, and thereby perhaps finally confirming the oncogenic properties of the virus.

Table 2. Criteria for viral carcinogenesis

1. Infection precedes development of tumour
2. Tumour cells should contain virus-specific antigens or particles
3. Tumour cells in culture could produce the virus
4. Virus should transform normal cells in culture or induce tumour in animals
5. Eradication of the virus should reduce tumour incidence

References

Beasley RP, Hwang LY (1984) Hepatocellular carcinoma and hepatitis B virus. Semin Liver Dis 4: 113–121

Bréchot C, Lugassy C, Dejean A, Pontisso P, Thiers V, Berthelot B, Tiollais B (1984) Hepatitis B virus DNA in infected human tissues. In: Vijas GN, Dienstag JL, Hoofnagle JH (eds) Viral hepatitis and liver disease. Grune & Stratton, New York, p. 395

Bréchot C, Degos F, Lugassy C, Thiers V, Zafrne S, Franco D, Bismuth H, Trepo C, Benhamon TP, Wands J, Isselbacher K, Tiollais P, Berthelot P (1985) Hepatitis B virus DNA in patients with chronic liver disease and negative tests for hepatitis B surface antigen. N Engl J Med 312: 270–273

Gerber MA, Thung SN (1985) Biology of disease. Molecular and cellular pathology of hepatitis B. Lab Invest 52: 572–590

Kew MC (1984) The possible etiologic role of the hepatitis B virus in hepatocellular carcinoma: evidence from South Africa. In: Chisari FV (ed) Advances in hepatitis research. Masson, New York, pp 203–215

Kew MC, Popper H (1984) Relationship between hepatocellular carcinoma and cirrhosis. Semin Liver Dis 4: 136–146

Sherman M, Shafritz DA (1984) Hepatitis B virus and hepatocellular carcinoma: molecular biology and mechanistic considerations. Semin Liver Dis 4: 98–112

Suzuki K, Uchida T, Horiuchi R, Shikata T (1985) Localization of hepatitis B surface and core antigens in human hepatocellular carcinoma by immunoperoxidase methods. Cancer 56: 321–327

Immunization Against Hepatitis B

A.J. ZUCKERMAN[1]

1 Plasma-Derived Vaccines

Hepatitis B surface antigen in the form of 22-nm spherical particles (and tubular forms) is excess virus coat protein. Guidelines for the preparation of the 22-nm spherical particles (and their separated polypeptides) derived from the plasma of asymptomatic human carriers were suggested by the WHO Expert Committee on Viral Hepatitis in 1977, and the proposed requirements for the 22-nm hepatitis B particle vaccine were published by the WHO Expert Committee on Biological Standardization in 1981 and revised in 1983. Such preparations have been tested for safety and protective efficacy, and many clinical studies in several million individuals with the plasma-derived vaccine have demonstrated the immunogenicity, high protective efficacy and safety of the currently licensed preparations meeting WHO requirements (Deinhardt and Zuckerman 1985).

Polypeptide vaccines, derived from the surface antigen from any source, have several advantages, which include precise biochemical characterization, exclusion of genetic material of viral origin, exclusion of host or donor-derived substances and enhanced potency. A polypeptide vaccine in micellar form has been developed in London. This preparation has been tested for safety and efficacy and has been shown to have enhanced immunogenecity. Clinical trials are in progress.

2 Vaccines Prepared by rDNA Techniques

The applications of recombinant DNA technology permit the isolation, purification and selective amplification of almost any individual segment of DNA from practically any organism in convenient biological systems such as bacteria, yeast, or any other cell including mammalian cells (Zuckerman 1985a,b).

Recombinant DNA techniques have been used for expressing hepatitis B surface antigen and core antigen in prokaryotic cells (*E. coli* and *B. subtilis*) and in eukaryotic cells, (*S. cerevisiae*). The yeast-derived vaccines are now under clinical trial. These studies have established the nucleotide sequence of hepatitis B DNA and the organization of the viral genome. The genome contains four major polypeptide "reading frames". The S gene codes for a protein of molecular weight 25,000 which resembles closely in

---

1 London School of Hygiene and Tropical Medicine, University of London, London, United Kingdom

Viral Hepatitis, ed. by F. Callea et al.
© Springer-Verlag Berlin Heidelberg 1986

predicted sequence the non-glycosylated major hepatitis B surface antigen polypeptide (p25) identified by electrophoretic analysis of 22-nm antigen particles purified from plasma of infected individuals. Another "reading frame", the C gene, codes for the 21,000 molecular weight viral core polypeptide. The third "reading frame", the putative polymerase P gene, overlaps the S gene, and the fourth "reading frame" is designated as X.

A contiguous upstream region of the open "reading frame" for the S region is termed the pre-surface or pre-S region. A 35 kilo-Dalton (dK) protein is partially encoded by the pre-S gene and mediates the binding or interaction of hepatitis B surface antigen and polyalbumin. Studies are in progress to determine whether the product of pre-S plays a part in protective immunization.

There are also preliminary observations which suggest that antibody to the core antigen (anti-core), and perhaps more probably antibody to the e antigen (anti-e) may provide at least partial protection against infection. Core antigen has been expressed in high titre in *E. coli*, and studies are in progress to establish whether antibodies to the core antigen enhance protection or reduce the severity of infection in experimentally infected chimpanzees.

3 Hybrid Vaccinia Virus Vaccines

Potential live vaccines using recombinant vaccinia viruses have been constructed for hepatitis B, and also for Herpes simplex, rabies and other viruses. Foreign viral DNA is introduced into the vaccinia DNA by construction of chimaeric genes. This is accomplished by homologous recombination in cells, since the large size of the genome of vaccinia virus (185,000 base pairs) precludes in vitro gene insertion. A chimaeric gene consisting of vaccinia virus promoter sequences ligated to the coding sequence for the desired foreign protein is flanked by vaccinia virus DNA in a plasmid vector. The hepatitis B surface antigen made by vaccinia virus recombinant was similar or identical in its polypeptide composition, buoyant density, sedimentation rate and antigenecity to material obtained from the plasma of hepatitis B carriers.

The recloned vaccinia virus containing hepatitis B surface antigen coding sequences was used to vaccinate rabbits with the production of typical vaccinia lesions in the skin and high titres of hepatitis B surface antibody in the circulation. Preliminary studies in chimpanzees indicated the feasibility of using a recombinant vaccinia virus. The vaccinated chimpanzees had a secondary antibody response when challenged intravenously with live hepatitis B virus of a heterologous subtype with a mild inapparent infection characterized by seroconversion to surface antibody and hepatitis B anti-core. Although the chimpanzees had little or no circulating surface antibody after vaccination when the recombinant vaccinia was growing in the skin, they were immunologically "primed". As a result the chimpanzees had a brisk and sustained antibody response, presumably due to newly synthesized surface antigen after challenge with live hepatitis B virus. IgG surface antibody and the anti-a responses were detected early, which is consistent with the anamnestic nature of the response.

At present, however, there is no accepted laboratory marker of attenuation or of virulence of vaccinia virus for man, not only in the host directly inoculated with the virus, but also after several passages in the same species. Alterations in the genome of vaccinia virus which are concomitant with the selection of recombinants may alter the virulence of the virus. It has been noted that interruption of the thymidine kinase gene of the virus by insertion of foreign DNA reduced its virulence for mice. Nevertheless, changes in host range or tissue tropism of vaccinia viruses may occur as a result of their genetic modification, and these could be caused by changes in the virus envelope as a result of the incorporation of gene products of the foreign viral genes inserted into the vaccinia virus.

The advantages of vaccinia virus recombinant as a vaccine include low cost, ease of administration by multiple pressure or by the scratch technique, vaccine stability, long shelf-life, and the use of polyvalent antigens. The known adverse reactions with vaccinia virus vaccines are well documented, and their incidence and severity must be carefully weighed against the adverse reactions associated with existing vaccines which a new recombinant vaccine might replace. There are also reports of spread of current strains of vaccinia virus to contacts and this may present problems.

4 Chemically Synthesized Hepatitis B Vaccines

The development of chemically synthesized polypeptide vaccines offers many advantages in attaining the ultimate goal of producing chemically uniform, safe and cheap viral immunogens to replace many current vaccines which often contain large quantities of irrelevant microbial antigenic determinants, proteins and other material additional to the essential immunogen required for the induction of a protective antibody. The preparation of antibodies against viral proteins using fragments of chemically synthesized peptides mimicking viral amino acid sequences is now a possible and attractive alternative approach in immunoprophylaxis. Successful mimicking of determinants of HBsAg using chemically synthesized peptides has been reported by several groups of investigators, both in linear forms and as cyclical peptides. Peptides have been synthesized which retain biological function and appropriate secondary structure, even though they have a limited sequence homology with the natural peptide or are much smaller.

Studies have been carried out recently by Brown et al. (1984), using a chemically synthetic peptide in a linear and in a cyclical polypeptide I of hepatitis B surface antigen. The synthetic antigens and the native polypeptide complex p23-gp28 purified from hepatitis B surface antigen (anti-HBs) in human sera. The levels and affinity of anti-HBs produced by healthy persons after immunization with the licensed plasma-derived hepatitis B vaccine were studied, using three antigens. The results showed that the antibody affinity increased progressively throughout the period of immunization, but the pattern of affinity maturation varied according to the peptide used as an antigen. The majority of individuals showed a significant rise in antibody affinity after the third (booster) dose of vaccine given at 6 months. The use of chemically synthetic peptides thus allows for the first time a quantitative and qualitative assessment of antibody responses to hepatitis B vaccine.

These studies also confirmed that selected peptides corresponding to relevant epitopes of hepatitis B surface antigen may be useful as synthetic hepatitis B vaccines.

References

Brown SE, Howard CR, Zuckerman AJ, Steward MW (1984) Affinity of antibody responses in man to hepatitis B vaccine determined with synthetic peptides. Lancet 2: 184–187

Deinhardt F, Zuckerman AJ (1985) Immunization against hepatitis B. Report on a WHO meeting. J Med Virol 17 (in press)

Zuckerman AJ (1984) Who should be immunised against hepatitis B? Br Med J 289: 1243–1244

Zuckerman AJ (1985a) Subunit, recombinant and syntherit hepatitis B vaccines. Microbiol Sci 2: 129–138

Zuckerman AJ (1985b) New hepatitis B vaccines (1985) Br Med J 290: 492–496

Summary

H. POPPER[1]

The comprehensive presentations on selected topics offered a panorama of the present status of our knowledge of viral hepatitis. Brescia was the proper site, not only because of its historical beauty, but also because of the high number of HBsAg carrier in Lombardy, 150,000 among about 9 million. The HBsAg carrier rate in Italy at large seems to be around 2%. As in any summary of an interesting meeting, two questions arise: (a) what was new in the presentations? and (b) what do we want to know in the future? Of the many important contributions, those of the three Italian authors were outstanding.

As reviewed by an interested observer who, however, is a dilettante in many aspects, these points can be listed:

1. The clinical presentation and evolution of viral hepatitis (VH) remain an interesting problem to which a series of observations have been presented. Pearls of wisdom, both clinical and histologic, will be listed here. The extrahepatic manifestations have been emphasized, particularly of hepatitis B, many of them caused by immune complexes. Their local formation is responsible for the nephrosis which, in turn, may be a rare cause of intractable ascites; 1% of Guillain-Barre syndrome are accompanied by hepatitis B. The syndrome, however, seldom is associated with aplastic anemia, found sometimes with viral hepatitis. The question of chronicity of VH and evolution to cirrhosis was particularly illuminated by the pathologic presentation, excellent reviews of our present knowledge. The big germinative centers, as B lymphocyte zones, in hepatitis NANB contrast with the low antibody response in this disease. In such zones of the portal tracts, the dendritic reticulum cells are found which are in contact with immune complexes; they differ from the interdigitating cells in the T zone on the periphery of the tracts, that means the area of piecemeal necrosis for which here the name "interface hepatitis" was proposed. Active connective tissue septa rich in segmented leukocytes were distinguished from passive septa resulting from confluent necrosis. Investigations in animal models facilitate the study of the evolution of the disease, which is accelerated in them; they also permit, better than in man, a histologic differentiation of the several types of virus infection and with it throw light on their pathogenesis. For instance, in hepatitis A virus (HAV)-infected marmosets, the virus was demonstrated in hepatocytes and bile canaliculi before actual necrosis set in, which suggests that the latter reflects a subsequent immunologic reaction. However, the fact that steroids in such marmoset infections accentuated the necrosis would rather be in keeping with

---

1 The Stratton Laboratory for the Study of Liver Diseases, Mount Sinai School of Medicine of the City University of New York, New York, 10029, USA

Viral Hepatitis, ed. by F. Callea et al.
© Springer-Verlag Berlin Heidelberg 1986

a cytotoxic potential of HAV. The question of evolution of the chronic forms of VH, that means B and non-A, non-B, still requires elucidation, including their geographical variations and social aspects. This includes the role of the "healthy" HBsAg carrier state, in which HBsAg-loaded hepatocytes may be the only significant histologic abnormality. The time and mode of transition of this carrier state to cirrhosis and HCC are indeed not known. In Africa and the Far East the state seems to mainly result from perinatal and infancy infections, with ground-glass cells observed as early as at 4 years of age (Hsu et al., in press), while in the industrial countries it usually develops after adult HBV infection.

2. Delta virus (HDV) infection received major attention, not only because of its discovery in nearby Turin, but also because of the overriding significance which it is gradually acquiring in the appreciation of HV at large. The HDV-RNA, having only 1.75 kilobases, is thus translated into very few proteins only. The distribution of the disease is peculiar, and an unusual variant with a characteristic histologic picture (microsteatosis associated with granular eosinophilic necrosis) accounts for Santa Marta and Labrea fevers in northern South America and in the Amazon river basin. The relation of this form to the common HDV infections is so far not clear. Epidemics are best reflected in the South American outbreaks, endemic frequency is seen at this time particularly in Arabian and possibly other Mediterranean regions and, peculiarly, in the Sowjet Union. Finally, high risk groups are drug addicts and polytransfused persons (e.g., hemophiliacs), less so homosexuals. A characteristic of HDV seems its tendency to geographical migration, the causes of which are not established; the experimental infection of woodchucks raises the possibility of animal reservoirs.

The spread of HDV infection is horizontal between family members and not vertical, as that of HBV. There seems to be some competition between HBV and HDV. Coinfection with HBV and HDV is usually a mild disease, although serum HBV-DNA was found in 31% of the cases. It hardly differs from HBV infection alone; fatal massive necrosis develops, although rarely. It is usually followed by immunity to HBV and HDV, and a carrier state for both is questioned. By contrast, superinfection has much higher mortality, although serum HBV-HDV was found in only 12%. Usually, HDV and HBV markers are present for a long time, particularly in anti-e-positive cases in which the tendency to chronicity is higher than in e-positive patients. Thus, overall mortality in 3-year follow-ups in HBV-DNA infections is three times higher than in pure HBV infections. In diagnosis, hybridization of serum HDV-RNA with cDNA is moving from a research to a routine technique superior to the demonstration of serum antigen (HDAg), since it prevails also longer in the blood than HDAg or the characteristic particles, especially in chronic disease. Both HBV-DNA and HDV-RNA may be in serum, for instance in drug addicts, especially with recent hepatitis and with impaired immunity. Prevention of HDV infections is difficult, particularly since coinfection is hard to evaluate. Control also is not easy. It depends on diagnosis. A specific vaccine is not yet on the horizon, but antiviral treatment with alpha-interferon has become promising, since it reduces at least temporarily serum HDV-RNA, together with a decline in the activities of the aminotransferases; this response has been also found in HBV-DNA-negative patients.

3. The tissue distribution of the various viral markers and the relation to serum markers reveal new vistas, particularly since in situ hybridization has become possible and now can even be carried out in paraffin sections (Rijntjes et al. 1985), in which also oncogen protein products (Jagirdar et al. 1985) or laminin have been visualized. HBV-DNA in the cytoplasm, presumably single-stranded and in more than 100 copies per cell, is seldom observed simultaneously with HBcAg in the same hepatocyte. It is not related to the e/anti-e status and seems to be associated with episomal HBV replication and hepatocellular injury (Burrel et al. 1984; Blum et al. 1983). HBV-DNA may be found in the serum in apparently healthy persons. It is sometimes seen even in the absence of HBsAg antigen but presence of anti-core antibodies. Its absence, however, can be considered a reliable sign of lack of infectivity. Immunocytochemical analysis permits the establishment of the relation of viral proteins to each other, to serum markers, and to the clinical evolution. A new observation is HBcAg in the cytoplasm of typical ground-glass hepatocytes which need not exhibit HBsAg. Such cytoplasmic core antigen, focally or diffuse, reflecting synthesis in the endoplasmic reticulum before packing, is considered an indication of aggressivity. A peculiar subgroup emerged in which cytoplasmic core antigen is associated with HBV-DNA and e antibody in the serum and indicates clinical severity of the disease; the combination of serum HBV-DNA with anti-e has been reported before and because of the ongoing viral replication, this condition should not be treated with steroids. Also combination of hepatocellular delta and core antigens speaks for a more severe disease status. Finally, membranous HBsAg in hepatocytes has long elicited arguments. Here it was reported that its significance depends on the amount and distribution of the simultaneous core antigen as well as of HLA-I's on the hepatocytes. Thus, hybridization of nucleic acids in serum and hepatocytes, combined with immunocytochemical visualization of viral antigens, now greatly carried out by Italian investigators, might enlighten the evolution of VH, particularly B.

4. Relatively little was added to the fascinating problems of *molecular biology of the hepatitis viruses*, a field which is rapidly progressing as promoters as well as enhancers and cis and trans acting factors are being unraveled and the life cycle of HBV is being recognized. For example, reference was barely made to the localization of HBV-DNA in cells other than hepatocytes, particularly in the lymphoid system. There, HBV-DNA may be in both free episomal and in integrated forms (Elfassi et al. 1983; Pontisso et al. 1984) and also in pancreatic cells, to conclude from observations in Hepadna viruses (Tagawa et al. 1985). To this point it was mentioned that lymphocytes of woodchucks also contain viral DNA, but the significance of this localization as either initial site in infection or as depot in chronicity was not elaborated on.

5. *The antibody response* is of major significance in viral clearance or protection and with it in vaccination but also in creation of hepatocellular injury by cellular immunity. The new monoclonal antibody techniques have clarified both the role of antibodies and the nature of the antigens. Viral antibodies may be protecting, binding, neutralizing, blocking or suppressing viral replication, with cytolysis the result of lymphocytic attack on cellular antigens. In acute hepatitis B, neutralization of the virus by binding to the SH bridge of dimers of HBsAg proteins or to the pre-s proteins may be important; it may occur independently of the proteins' glycosylation; the binding to pre-s$_1$ may be neutralizing and that to pre-s$_2$ may raise the immune response to another protein. Pre-s$_2$ represents the site binding to polymerized albumin (Offensperger et al. 1985), which was here reported not to bind to polyalbumin in woodchucks. The humoral antibodies may be IgM anti-c, anti-e, anti-s. Anti-s seems not to block,

but each of its epitopes may have another capacity. Anti-e apparently suppresses viral replication. In cytolysis viral antigens in the cell membrane are the targets of both allogenic-restricted T killer cells and of not restricted antibody-dependent cytotoxicity. Anti-s neither blocks the former by antigen binding nor serves in the latter. Anti-c seems not to block in vitro but to serve in the latter, while anti-e acting on a component of the c antigen (free of its RNA-binding site) seems to fulfill both functions. In vivo IgG anti-c directed against a specific epitope delays the removal of infected hepatocytes, and such monoclonal antibodies injected with an HBV load into chimpanzees produce a prolonged infection. Additional studies should confirm many of these effects in vivo, so important in understanding pathogenesis of chronic hepatitis.

6. In *the mechanism of the hepatocytic injury*, HDV and the common non-A, non-B agents seem to exert mainly a cytotoxic effect (Popper 1983), while in HBV infections lymphocytotoxicity is the important factor. The unsettled question as to HAV was mentioned before. In HBV-associated injury, action of interferon was reported here to be a key factor in pathogenesis.

Alpha-interferon (lymphoblastoid) formed in hepatocytes or administered has four hepatic effects, namely (1) it inhibits viral replication by inducing the specific 2-5A synthetase, (2) it increases HLA-I expression of hepatocytes, (3) the hepatocellular genome was here reported to contain an interferon-sensitive sequence necessary for induction of antiviral and HLA proteins; this sequence is homologous to sequences in HBV (consensus); and (4) interferon accounts for some clinical symptoms of hepatitis. In the chronicity of HBV infection three potentially alpha-interferon related mechanisms may be important: (1) In the initial adult HBsAg carrier state, which follows less than 10% of acute HBV infections, the response to anti-c and anti-e is normal, but endogenous interferon production is impaired. This favors the spread of the HBV and also inhibits HLA-I expression on the infected hepatocytes, resulting in impaired removal of infected cells by cytotoxic T cells; in this situation, therapeutic administration of interferon is most effective. (2) By contrast, in later carrier states the integration of HBV into the host genome may take place in the previously mentioned homologous interferon therapy-responsive sequence of the genome, rendering these hepatocytes insensitive to interferon; on discontinuation of interferon, HBV may spread again from these to other hepatocytes, which explains the common response to interferon therapy, namely, temporary suppression of HBV replication. (3) In infants, acute HBV infection is almost invariably followed by a carrier state, which was here explained by the transplacental passage of IgG anti-core, which delays by blocking of the antigen the action of the cytotoxic T cells, despite their HLA expression; therefore, therapeutic interferon has no effect. These mechanisms complement the several others commonly considered.

7. Antibody responses are, of course, crucial in HBV *vaccination*. Not only are epitopes of the several HBsAg proteins of importance, but possibly, besides the pre-s, core antigen in the vaccine may contribute to postvaccination immunity. Several important vaccination-related questions include (1) the priority of persons to receive it, (2) the schedule, (3) the duration of immunity, with revaccination considered 3 or 7 years later, (4) the management of poor or non-responders, and (5) the type of the vaccine, to be judged by (a) immunogenicity, (b) effectiveness, and (c) safety. By now, several millions of plasma-derived vaccinations have been performed. Among second-genera-

tion vaccines, those made by recombinant techniques, yeast vaccine is now in wide use. Constructions such as using the vaccinia virus as carrier are attractive because of relatively low expenses and the long experience with its vaccination. The third generation, the synthetic vaccines, might be cheaper because they might require only a limited number of amino acids as linear or cyclic peptides after the crucial immunogenic epitope is identified. As by-product, a synthetic vaccine permits not only measurement of the amount but also qualitative assessment of its affinity, which also seems to rise after repeated doses and particularly after the booster dose. Anti-idiotype antibody vaccines are so far only a glint in our eyes (Kennedy et al. 1984).

8. Antiviral therapy continues to result in an only temporary depression of replication in chronic hepatitis, particularly e-positive, and combinations of interferon with adenine arabinoside therapy continue to be tried. Therapy, particularly with interferon, is especially ineffective in homosexuals (and probably also drug addicts) because of their immune suppression, particularly if antibodies to HTLV-III are present, even without clinical symptoms of AIDS. Similar ineffectiveness has been found in the treatment of delta-infected drug addicts. Ara-A is preferable over interferon in Orientals because of the mechanisms previously listed. The fact that, in western and northern Europe and in United States, drug addicts and homosexuals, both with potentially altered immune status, represent the bulk of chronic HBV infections, might explain the difference from other countries in disease evolution and response to therapy, for instance to steroids and antivirals.

9. The relation of HBV infection to hepatocellular carcinoma is a most significant problem, in view of the wide spread of HBsAg-positive HCC throughout the world, with supposedly about 250,000 deaths per year (WHO, 1983). The vast majority are in Subsaharan Africa and the Far East, while the incidence is relatively low in the industrialized world. It was here well reviewed from various viewpoints, particularly that of prospective versus retrospective epidemiology. The question of the carcinogenicity of the virus appears to be resolved, to judge from the reported experiences with the woodchuck hepatitis virus, which in laboratory-infected animals produced hepatocellular carcinoma without exposure to a co-carcinogen; a role of a promoting factor is, however, not excluded. Integration of viral HBV-DNA into the host genome can be considered as inititation, and possibly further changes of the DNA, both integrated viral and host sequences (Rogler and Summers 1984; Rogler et al. 1985), may represent promotion. Questions not resolved include (1) the role of cirrhosis, which may be a promoting factor, and the time points of its development, (2) type of integration and its modifications, (3) identification of the promoting factors, and (4) possibly antagonism between HBV replication and integration, which enters into indications of antiviral therapy, which preferably should be carried out before integration has become extensive. The fascination with HCC is, of course, the possibility that HBV vaccination may in the future eliminate one of the most common fatal malignancies of mankind. Just as the relation between smoking and lung cancer was proven by the decline of the tumour's incidence associated with reduction of smoking, an eventual conspicuous reduction of HCC incidence after vaccination may become the most convincing proof of the causal relation.

Relatively little was said about *hepatitis non-A, non-B,* for which reliable markers still do not exist. In contrast to the epidemic form with the epidemiology of hepatitis A and lack of chronicity, the common form with the epidemiology of hepatitis B is, as was again pointed out, now the most common posttransfusion hepatitis, at least in the industrialized world; regrettable, in other areas, screening of blood has not yet completely eliminated HBV infection. To reduce NANB infection, screening of blood by elevated activities of aminotransferases is popular in Europe but not in the United States. By contrast elimination of anti-c-positive blood is discouraged, not only because it need not detect concomitant NANB infection, but also because it may reduce protection against HBV which has escaped even sophisticated screening techniques. Whether heat treatment eliminates all forms of NANB is not settled. The responsible agent remains the key problem in the disease. Although its histologic expressions seem to differ from HBV infections (Popper 1983), there are interesting but so far not confirmed observations of integrated HBV-DNA in the absence of serum markers (Marcellin et al. 1985) and of demonstration by monoclonal antibodies of HBV-related hepatopathogenic variants (Wands et al. 1985), which might represent human types of Hepadna viruses.

In conclusion, the meeting in Brescia was attended by an interested, indeed enthusiastic audience, which raises the hope of a similar reception of the book by the readers. Both audience and readership should be grateful to AVIS (Italian Association of Blood Donors), which celebrated its 50th anniversary, and to the organizing committee, particularly Professor M. Zorzi and Dr. F. Callea, but also to their advisor, Professor V.J. Desmet of Leuven. Seldom have the problems of viral hepatitis been presented so effectively.

References

Blum H, Stowring L, Figus A, Montgomery C, Haase A, Vyas G (1983) Detection of HBV DNA in hepatocytes, bile duct epithelium and vascular elements in in situ hybridization. Proc Natl Acad Sci USA 80: 6685–6688

Burrel CJ, Gowans EJ, Rowland R, Hall P, Jilbert AR, Marmion BP (1984) Correlation between liver histology in markers of hepatitis B virus replication in infected patients: a study by in situ hybridization. Hepatology 4: 20–24

Elfassi E, Romet-Lemonne J, Essex M, McLane M, Haseltine W (1983) Evidence of extrachromosomal forms of HBV DNA in a bone marrow culture obtained from a patient recently infected with a hepatitis B virus. Proc Natl Sci USA 81: 3526–3528

Hsu HC, Chang MH, Lin YH, Beasley RP, Hwang LY, Lee CY, Popper H (1986) Hepatic histopathologic observations and hepatitis B virus (HBV) antigens in children with vertical transmission of HBV by asymptomatic chronic carrier mothers. Hepatology (in press)

Jagirdar J, Nonomura A, Patil J, Paronetto F (1985) Activated ras oncogene p21 expression in hepatocellular carcinoma (HCC) and HBsAg-positive liver cells. Hepatology 5: 435

Kennedy RC, Melnick JL, Dreesman GR (1984) Antibody to hepatitis B virus induced by injecting antibodies to the idiotype. Science 223: 930–931

Marcellin P, Pasquinelli C, Belghitti J, Tiollais P, Brechot C, Benhamou JP (1985) Is HBV infection the cause of HBsAg-negative chronic active hepatitis in the Maghreb? Hepatology 5: 969

Offensperger W, Wahl S, Neurath AR, Price P, Strick N, Kent SBH, Christman JK, Acs G (1985) Expression in *Escherichia coli* of a cloned DNA sequence encoding the pre-s$_2$ region of hepatitis B virus. Proc Natl Acad Sci USA 82: 7540–7544

Pontisso P, Poon M, Tiollais P, Brechot C (1984) Detection of HBV DNA in mononuclear blood cells. Br Med J 288: 1563–1566

Popper H (1983) Concluding remarks. In: Verme G, Bonino F, Rizzetto M (eds) Viral hepatitis and
    delta infection. Liss, New York, pp 397–410
Report of a W.H.O. scientific group (1983) Chairman; Zuckerman AJ. Lancet 1: 463–465
Rijntjes PJM, Van Dithuhuijsen Th JM, Van Loon AM, Van Haelst UJGM, Bronkhorst FB, Yap SH
    (1985) Hepatitis B virus DNA detected in formalin-fixed liver specimens and its relation to
    serologic markers and histopathologic features in chronic liver disease. Am J Pathol 120: 411–
    418
Rogler CE, Summers J (1984) Cloning and structural analysis of integrated woodchuck hepatitis
    virus sequences from a chronically infected liver. J Virol 50: 832–837
Rogler CE, Sherman M, Su CY, Shafritz DA, Summers J, Shows TB, Henderson A, Kew M (1985)
    Deletion in chromosome 11p associated with a hepatitis B integration site in hepatocellular car-
    cinoma. Science 230: 319–322
Tagawa M, Omata M, Yokosuka O, Uchiumi K, Imazeki F, Okuda H (1985) Early events in duck
    hepatitis B virus infection. Sequential appearance of viral deoxyribonucleic acid in the liver,
    pancreas, kidney and spleen. Gastroenterology 89: 1224–1229
Wands JR, Fujita YK, Isselbacher KJ, Degott C, Schellekens H, Dazza MC, Tiollais P, Brechot C
    (1985) Identification and transmission of hepatitis B virus (HBV) related variants. Hepatology
    5: 1054

Subject Index

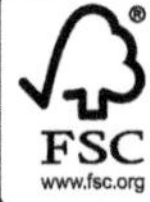